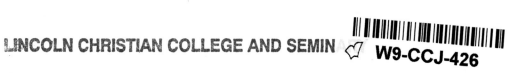

Praise for

BODY BY GOD

The Owner's Manual for Maximized Living

by Dr. Ben Lerner

We were very pleased to have Dr. Ben Lerner associated with the US World and Olympic wrestling teams. Ben's feedback during the team's training and preparation made my job, as a coach, much easier. Ben's work ethic and energy put him in a success level of his own. Now, with *Body By God,* Ben is enabling others to achieve success by providing a complete blueprint that anyone, not just elite athletes, can follow.

—Bruce Burnett
U.S. World & Olympic Wrestling Team Coach (1992, 1996, 2000)
Head Wrestling Coach, United States Naval Academy

In building a career and a family, we have learned how important it is to stay strong—from the inside out. The key to a truly fulfilling life is to strengthen yourself physically, nutritionally, spiritually, and mentally. The principles Dr. Ben outlines in his book, *Body by God,* are simple, smart, and easy to apply to your life.

—Grant and Tamia Hill
NBA All Star and 4-Time Grammy Nominee

As a minister and professional musician for more than 15 years, I have struggled in the attempt to secure a healthy, nutritional lifestyle while traveling more than 150 days out of the year. Thank God for Dr. Ben Lerner! His "Body by God" principles, derived in part by the greatest "handbook for living" ever written, the Bible, have helped me to not only feel better physically, but to remember that God Himself desires me to be strong, well, and full of life (John 10:10, Jer. 29:11). This is no fad diet, this is a lifestyle—a revelation of health, hope, and happiness.

—Andy Chrisman
Founding Member of Christian Music Group 4HIM
Minister of Music and Worship, Celebrate Family Church, Celebration, FL

The *Body by God* concept that your body is by God and for God totally fits into my game plan, on and off the field. The exercise and nutrition program in the *Owner's Manual for Maximized Living* will help me stay healthy and running for a long time. Doctor Ben gives great information about stress and time management, too, which will help me with two of the most important areas of my life: (1) Experiencing a powerful relationship with God; and (2) Maintaining a strong family life.

—Shaun Alexander
University of Alabama All-SEC and SEC Offensive Player of the Year
and NFL's Seattle Seahawks Star Running Back

More than any other time in our history we are living longer, and the advances in science tell us that in the next decade or so there will be breakthroughs that will bring the average lifespan up to about a century. Sadly, while we are living longer many are living with more illnesses and diseases that are preventable or treatable. We need an approach to the life and the body that is rooted and grounded in the way our bodies were made to live. Of the many health care professionals I have been privileged to be associated with over the years, I have come to deeply appreciate and value the work of my dear friend and colleague Dr. Ben Lerner and his *Body by God* approach to health, wholeness, and well-being. Dr. Ben's practical advice and personal life experience—combined with running one of the top 2 largest and most successful chiropractic centers on the planet, precisely because of his *Body by God* approach—make this book invaluable to anyone truly interested in getting more years out of life and more life out of their years. In a day when so many drug therapies have numbed us to the real root causes of our physical conditions, this book offers a "take responsibility for your life and health" hands-on approach to becoming everything you were intended to become. You want to get in shape? You want to be well and feel great from head to toe and from inside out? You want to be fully alive with every step and breath you take? *Body by God* isn't just a book to read once . . . it is a book to live by for the rest and best of your life!

—Mark J. Chironna, Ph.D.
Overseer of The Master's Touch International Church in Orlando. FL

I met Dr. Ben Lerner at the USA wrestling training camps prior to the 1996 Centennial Olympic Games in Atlanta. Dr. Ben's time spent with the athletes, his own experience in weight management and stress control, as well as his strong belief in God proved to be a great asset to the team. The physical and mental health of our athletes was a major factor in the US team's success in the Olympic Games and our first Gold Medal Team Championship with all major countries in attendance.

—**Joe Seay**
USA Wrestling Team Head Coach, 1996 Olympic Games
National Wrestling Hall of Fame Distinguished Member

For both better and for worse, science and technology relentlessly continues to revolutionize our lives at a dizzying and confusing pace. As a result, there is a mounting need for simplicity, clarity, and truth. The best resolution for uncertainty is to understand and draw upon principles that stand the test of time and an ever-changing knowledge base. Recent history has shown us that often we must unlearn what we once thought was truth. But, in fact, it is a reminder that there is only one timeless Truth. It is within this context that Dr. Ben Lerner provides a much-needed lens through which to clearly view and maximize our health and well-being. With so much disease and stress and a significant lack of joy and peace in our lives, we forget that health, not sickness, is our natural created state. *Body By God* is an owner's manual to both remind us of that fact and to teach us how to create a context in which our body, mind, and soul can thrive as God intended.

—**Mark J. Adams, ND, M.S.**
Doctor of Naturopathic Medicine
and Well-Care Management Specialist (Seattle)

When I met Dr. Ben two years ago, I was about to give up my lifelong passion for sailing due to severe neck pain. Within weeks of following his plan for diet and exercise I was back aboard without pain and with incredible energy. *Body by God* puts it all together and provides the details necessary to understand the reasons behind his inspired advice.

—**James A. Doran**
Stetson University

Dr. Ben Lerner has been a valuable asset for our elite USA Wrestling team athletes as they prepared for and participated in the World Championships and the Olympic Games. Dr. Ben volunteered his time and resources to help our athletes reach their optimal performance level. His contribution has been recognized as an integral asset to the team's success by both the athletes and the coaching staff.

—**Mitch Hull**
National Teams Director, USA Wrestling

Dr. Ben Lerner has written an incredibly comprehensive book titled *Body by God*. In it he addresses a full complement of information on the whole makeup of man.

Regarding our physical well-being, Dr. Ben gets right down where the rubber meets the road—the "how-to's" of what we should gravitate toward and what we should stay away from when it comes to natural health. With clarity and keen insight he establishes key principles on how to manage the issues of the soul—your mind, will, and emotions. Most importantly, Dr. Ben digs deeper still to uncover the "God Connection"—matters of the human heart and spirit that help us stay the course of total well-being through time and eternity.

This is not a breeze-through book! Take time to read, study, and digest its contents until your whole man—spirit, soul, and body—is fit for the Master's use.

—**Stephen Sumrall**
President, Lester Sumrall Evangelistic Association (LeSEA)

BODY BY GOD

BODY BY GOD

THE OWNER'S MANUAL FOR MAXIMIZED LIVING

DR. BEN LERNER

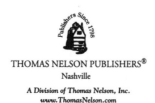

THOMAS NELSON PUBLISHERS®
Nashville

A Division of Thomas Nelson, Inc.
www.ThomasNelson.com

Published in Nashville, Tennessee, by Thomas Nelson, Inc.

In view of the complex, individual nature of health and fitness problems, this book, and the ideas, programs, procedures, and suggestions are not intended to replace the advice of trained medical professionals. All matters regarding one's health require medical supervision. A physician should be consulted prior to adopting any program or programs described in this book or any of the Body by God series. The author and publisher disclaim any liability arising directly or indirectly from the use of this book.

Unless otherwise noted, Scripture quotations are from the HOLY BIBLE: NEW INTERATIONAL VERSION®. Copyright © 1973, 1978, 1984 by International Bible Society. Used by permission of Zondervan Publishing House. All rights reserved.

Scripture quotations noted NKJV are from THE NEW KING JAMES VERSION. Copyright © 1979, 1980, 1982, Thomas Nelson, Inc., Publishers.

Scripture quotations noted NCV are from THE HOLY BIBLE, NEW CENTURY VERSION, copyright © 1987, 1988, 1991 by W Publishing, a Division of Thomas Nelson, Inc. Used by permission.

Author photos on book jacket were taken by Douglas Scaletta.

Exercise photos, as well as photos in the park, were taken by Thomas E. Naylor, Tom Naylor Photography, Celebration, Florida.

Library of Congress Cataloging-in-Publication Data

Lerner, Ben.
   Body by God : the owner's manual for maximized living / Ben Lerner.
      p. cm.
   ISBN 0-7852-6317-9
   1. Health—Religious aspects—Christianity. I. Title.
BT732.L45 2003
248.4—dc22   2003019725

Printed in the United States of America
05 06 07 QWM 7

The following doctors are all contributors and trusted providers of the science and principles found in this book. They are some of the most caring, God-serving, capable doctors of any kind in the world.

Arizona
Dr. Mitchell Borst
Dr. David Stender

California
Dr. Jeffery Ptak
Dr. Gavin Grant
Dr. Todd Royse
Dr. Jeff Gancas
Dr. Kenneth Moger

Colorado
Dr. Tom Bolan
Dr. Keppen Laszlo
Dr. Ty Johnson
Dr. Brent Berlener
Dr. Jason Keller
Dr. Brad Richardson

Florida
Dr. Patrick St. Germain
Dr. Mickey Cohen
Dr. Roger Romano
Dr. Dan Yachter
Dr. Erik Lerner
Dr. Tony Nalda
Dr. Tim Bassett
Dr. Daniel Barr
Dr. Dave Yachter

Dr. Dave Golinger
Dr. Greg Loman
Dr. Rich Lerner
Dr. Travis Wells

Georgia
Dr. Michael Huppert
Dr. Mark Domanski
Dr. Shoanmarie Seals

Idaho
Dr. Zane Sterling
Dr. Keith McKim

Indiana
Dr. Joel Feeman
Dr. Rob Schiffman

Iowa
Dr. Tom Schiltz

Kentucky
Dr. Lewis Misinay
Dr. Terry Harmon
Dr. Rick Hellmann

Louisiana
Dr. Patrick McNeil
Dr. Phillip Smith

Massachusetts
Dr. Tria Sykes
Dr. Allison Glass

Michigan
Dr. Mark McCullough

Minnesota
Dr. Brian Arvold
Dr. Peter Wurdemann

Nebraska
Dr. Linn Erickson

New Hampshire
Dr. Holly Ruocco

New Jersey
Dr. Brad Butler
Dr. Frank Berzanskis

New Mexico
Drs. Daniel &
    Barbara Bartel

New York
Dr. Tom Kovacs
Dr. Craig Fishel

North Carolina
Dr. Keith Helmendach

112455

Dr. Sonya Young
Dr. Megan Powell
Dr. John Hanna
Dr. Jeff Zitel

Ohio
Dr. Matt Pamer
Dr. Mackenzie Pamer
Dr. Dale Capela
Dr. Jonathan Snyder

Oklahoma
Dr. John Godfrey

Pennsylvania
Dr. Tom Horn
Dr. Jeremiah Schreiber
Dr. Ray Wisniewski

Texas
Dr. Rick Housewright

Washington
Dr. Deborah Adams
Dr. Ted Cunningham
Dr. Paul Reed

Canada
Dr. Terri Wells (Alberta)
Dr. Joel Bohemier
(Manitoba)

For more information on Body by God providers, Body by God products and services, and/or to contact Dr. Ben, visit www.thebodybygod.com.

CONTENTS

ABOUT
THE AUTHOR

Dr. Ben Lerner served as a U.S. Olympic team physician at the 1996 Atlanta Centennial Olympic Games and again at the 2000 Olympic games held in Sydney, Australia. He has trained and traveled with the 1995, '97, '98, and '99 Freestyle and Greco-Roman World Wrestling Teams, and his center for Maximized Living is one of the largest clinics in the world.

Through his own personal accomplishments with the U.S. Olympic wrestling teams, to those of his celebrity clients, including professional athletes, Dr. Ben Lerner is a corporate consultant who is a living testament to every life-altering page of this book, *Body by God: The Owner's Manual for Maximized Living.*

Dr. Ben's life experiences helped to shape his Body by God philosophy. He jokingly refers to himself as a victim of "Poor Genetic Syndrome," although it is plain to see that he is the picture of health. What does he mean by this?

Ben considered himself at a genetic disadvantage primarily due to the fact that the majority of people in his family were overweight, stressed out, and for the most part dead before the age of sixty. Accordingly, Dr. Ben felt the urgency to uncover a method of improving his mind, body, and spirit with the goal of looking good, enjoying life, and living longer. His journey to overcome what seemed to be a predisposition to poor health and a lackluster life is embodied in his teachings, seminars, and writing.

THE BODY BY GOD QUICK REFERENCE GUIDE

Where to Turn to See Some Changes Today!

Your Body by God Owner's Manual is broken up into five parts:

1. Maximizing Your Life
2. Fueling Your Body by God
3. Moving Your Body by God
4. Stress Management for Your Body by God
5. Time Management for Your Body by God

All of these together will bring you closer to a Life by God, which is the concluding section of this book. In it you will find the entire "Body by God 40-Day Plan."

> **IMPORTANT TIP:** If one part of the book interests you right now more than another, you can skip directly to that part.

The following is a quick reference guide to the different areas covered in *Body by God*. It will show you how you can begin getting results right away in the area or areas that interest you most.

Maximizing Your Life

Turn to page 21 and discover "The Four Rules of Olympic Success." These rules will show you how Olympians, who are the "best of the best of the best" have become so successful at such a high level. By duplicating some of their methods you, too, can become successful at most anything and at most any level.

Nutrition

To see quick results in your health and appearance and to start losing unwanted pounds right away, begin adding food from the "Food by God" list found on pages 48–51 and start reducing food from the "Food by Man" list found on page 55.

To see even quicker, more radical changes also follow the "Un-Diet Food Guide" found on pages 82–84. This unique guide is the premiere part of the nutrition section. The Un-Diet Food Guide tells you how much and what time of day you should eat your carbohydrates, proteins, and fats. You will see remarkable changes using the food guides even if you do not significantly change what types of food you are eating!

Exercise

To initiate, immediately, an incredibly effective, safe, fat-burning aerobic routine, turn to "Finding Your Aerobic Moving Zones" on page 152. This section will reveal to you what are your Fat Burning Zones while doing cardiovascular exercises and how to create your very own program.

For a brand new body in just weeks, in addition to creating your own fat-burning aerobic program, institute the Body by God "Quick Sets" resistance program. Quick Sets found on page 205 are a set of weight-lifting routines that show you how to get stronger, leaner muscles in workouts that last as little as three minutes.

Stress Management

Turn to page 240 and inaugurate your study of "The 10 Instructions for Peace by God." Reading this portion of the stress management part of your owner's manual will instantaneously begin reprogramming the way you look at, and react to, the stress in your life.

Time Management

Do you want to find out how you can feel as if you are doubling or even quadrupling the amount of time you have in a week? If so, turn to page 313 to see how to schedule your life and paint solid yellow lines around Time by God. This will help you commence putting your life back on track and give you the time to implement your new nutrition, exercise, and stress-management routines.

When using the Quick Reference Guide always keep in mind how important is each area of the Body by God; the Owner's Manual for Maximized Living is for reaching your God-given potential. Real prosperity can only be found by finding success in many areas of your lifestyle and not just one.

 CAUTION: BEFORE MAKING SIGNIFICANT CHANGES IN NUTRITIONAL HABITS OR BEGINNING NEW FORMS OF EXERCISE, ALWAYS CONSULT YOUR PHYSICIAN FIRST.

INTRODUCTION

Using Your Owner's Manual for Maximized Living

If life hasn't been working out, it's because you haven't read the manual.

If someone gives you a car, a computer, a watch, a TV, a DVD player, a board game, an electronic planner, or anything else that's complex, you need to read the owner's manual in order to learn how to use it, maintain it, fix it, and get maximum enjoyment and benefit from it.

If you do not read the manual, you usually end up utilizing only a small percentage of the potential these gifts have to offer. You never really learn how to operate them properly or even set the clock. When one of these toys or gadgets doesn't seem to work or breaks, it is typically not due to manufacturer error but because you, the owner, failed to read the manual.

You have been given the most awesome, divine, complex gift in the world: your body. If life has not been working out, it is not the fault of the manufacturer! Pains, dysfunctions, failures, and psychological and emotional breakdowns are most likely due to a failure to read the manual. Well, this is your manual! This book is the owner's manual for maximized living in your Body by God.

You are a Body by God (BBG) owner. God created you with the intention that you would have a prosperous journey filled with incredible health and outrageous happiness. So just as you familiarize yourself with owner's manuals for cars, stereos, watches, and computers, follow the guidelines in this book—your owner's manual—in order to get the most benefit, enjoyment, and longest use out of your BBG.

> **Man's ideas come and go, but God's clothes never go out of style.**

THE FAILURE OF HUMAN THINKING

The reason most health books and positive-mental-attitude programs fail to create any long-term success is that the information is only man's and little of it is God's. While human teachings and philosophies often can be good impersonators of God's wisdom, they are devoid of any real power. This "human wisdom" may bring what appears to be a certain level of success, but it will always be short-term. You'll never find what God intended for you by following the ways of man alone. A house built on only human wisdom is a foundationless house that will surely fall to the ground.

When you impose human will instead of God's will, a domino effect of actions and reactions is created that causes perpetual failure. While man's information may motivate you, make you feel good, or temporarily put you on a better track, human wisdom will not bring you the wholeness and richness you deserve. While you may feel good now, without God, sickness and despair are just waiting to rear their ugly heads.

The limitations of human thought are obvious. Every few years, new information comes to light that completely eliminates the old standards of thinking. No matter how much we humans think we know about ourselves and the world we live in, we eventually find out we are wrong. At some point, all of man's latest, greatest discoveries become obsolete. For example:

- *In Space Study:* Many times we have felt we knew all there was to know about certain regions of space, only to later discover a black hole and come upon masses of undiscovered stars and miles of uncharted territory.

- *In Medicine:* We have totally believed time and again that we knew how to treat certain illnesses, only to later find there were not only better treatments, but the old methods actually were quite damaging, delayed healing, or were even more deadly than the illness itself. Bloodletting, applying leeches, and drilling holes in the skull to let out evil demons were literally the premier medical procedures of their day.

- *In Health:* Years ago, smoking was actually recommended as a way to relax, and vitamins were believed by doctors to have no benefit and were thought to give you only "expensive urine." High-carbohydrate, low-protein, no-fat diets were recommended for a while, then no-carbohydrate, high-protein, high-fat diets, then a combination of both. (The Food Guide in the Food by God chapter of this book will set you straight on the right way to eat.)

- *In Athletics:* There was a time when athletes would not lift weights for fear it would impede their performance. Strength training has since totally transformed the world of sports.

- *In Life:* Clothing, travel, hairstyles, civil rights, computer technology, education, and hundreds of other elements of society are continuously being revolutionized so much so that if you look back even just a few months, the changes are astonishing.

A tremendous amount of what is accepted as truth or science today will tomorrow be found to be faulty or possibly even harmful. All human knowledge is temporary. There is always a higher level of understanding that shows man's wisdom to contain some level of ignorance.

The only existing permanent, flawless, and limitless wisdom comes from God. Only His thinking is genuine, always at its peak, always to build up, never to destroy, and always succeeds. In other words, *God's clothes never go out of style.*

Don't limit yourself by holding on to old, eventually outdated human discoveries. Seek only methods and ideas that come from sources or people who have sought God's unlimited wisdom—like those found in this book, your *Owner's Manual*—and not their own limited thought.

In *Body by God: The Owner's Manual for Maximized Living,* I have attempted to offer methods and ideas that not only make common sense, people sense, and scientific sense, they make God sense.

> As the heavens are higher than the earth, so are my ways higher than your ways and my thoughts than your thoughts. (Isa. 55:9)

PART ONE | MAXIMIZING YOUR LIFE

1 | THE BODY
BY GOD (BBG)

After nearly twenty years in the healthy, happy lifestyle world, taking care of tens of thousands of patients of all ages, and working with Olympic and professional athletes, I have discovered one elemental truth: *There is a creator of the human body and it is not me.* This understanding has helped me not to create but to lead more people toward a better appearance, healthier body, and more peaceful outlook on life than any other one thing I know.

The true, underlying principle of *Body by God* is the knowledge that if we took everything we know about how God designed and created the body, multiplied that knowledge by a trillion, and then added infinity, we still would not have even a glimpse of understanding what He has done. No person can make another. The body is not by man; the body is by God—which is really quite fortunate, if you think about it. The things man makes tend to wear out pretty quickly. If body parts were like answering machines, lightbulbs, and auto parts, you'd have to replace them several times a year. If your body were like a computer, it would become obsolete within months and needed to be upgraded, or possibly even discarded for a new one. Luckily for us, the Adam and Eve prototypes are still fully operational today, have never lost their value, and will never become obsolete.

God is not only the Producer; He is also the Executive Director. His power, which created all things, created you. His power is constantly on the job controlling, sustaining, healing, creating, and re-creating every part and system of your Body by God (BBG).

Your BBG is a miraculous gift that God has handed over to you for the relatively brief duration of your lifetime. Showing respect for your gift means showing respect and love for God. Unfortunately, for many this respect and love have been discarded and replaced by stress, inactivity, inadequate nutrition, and a tremendous amount of wasted time.

This irreverence for our bodies is made most evident by just looking at what people are willing to put in their mouths.

It has become the shocking nutritional truth that the most popular food in the world today is not known for its quality, its nutrient content, its geographical origin, or even its taste. Instead, it is known for its speed. It is literally called "fast food."

In fact, with all fast-food restaurants having drive-thru windows these days, service is faster than ever. We do not even have to get out of our vehicles anymore to eat. Now families can eat in vans, just as God intended . . . ?

Fueling your BBG with what is quickest, rather than what is best, damages your gift, keeps you from performing at your peak potential, and stops you from having the kind of reliable energy you need to best serve your Creator.

Your body is not your own! Your body is not only *by* God, it is *for* God, and it *is* God's. Everyone on earth was placed here with a mission from God. God chooses specific people to perform specific tasks for Him. For that task or mission to be fulfilled so that God's will may be done, you must stay inspired to take care of your BBG in a way that allows it to thrive and live up to its potential.

If you were high on crack cocaine, drunk from alcohol, or suffering with serious pain or illness, could you be successful in your occupation, relate well with others, or take good care of yourself? Obviously not! You would not be able to think clearly, you would be off mentally, and you would be physically tired.

This is an exaggerated version of what happens to you when you put the wrong food in your BBG, when you treat it improperly by never moving off your couch or away from your desk, and when you experience too much stress.

The toxins, chemicals, and unhealthy materials that exist in fast foods and other poor-quality foods, as well as the effects of stress and lack of movement, harmfully affect the mind and body. Rather than creating the more obvious and massive dysfunction brought about by cocaine use, alcohol use, or pain and illness, dietary poisons, anxiety, and inactivity more subtly irritate your system, affect your moods, cloud your mind, and rob your body of strength and health. As a result, your effectiveness, your relationship with others and God, and your length of time on this planet are negatively affected.

Sickness, disease, the pains of poor health, defective relationships, chronic failure, and persistent unhappiness are just the symptoms and side effects of not caring for your life the way God intended.

My goal for working with all of my patients and in writing this book is to move people toward taking care of themselves not just Dr. Ben's way or any other doctor's or author's way—but God's way.

I am looking to help you remember that your body is by God, for God, and is God's. Your Body by God is a gift from God. What you do with your BBG is your gift to Him.

> Know that the LORD is God. It is he who made us, and we are his; we are his people, the sheep of his pasture. (Ps. 100:3)

BODY BY GOD: NO ASSEMBLY REQUIRED

Man cannot make a body. Therefore, man cannot fix a body or truly determine its needs. God, on the other hand, can make a body and knows exactly what it requires at all times. Inside your Body by God is a symphony of thousands of functions and chemical reactions we know about, and endless ones only God knows about. All these functions and reactions happen at precisely the right time, at the right place, and for all the right reasons. Each moment of each day, the body is repairing tissue, creating new cells, and balancing billions of tiny little operating systems.

Because we have no idea what is really going on, all we can do is respect God's BBG, see its vast potential, appreciate its brilliance, and place no interference in its natural path. Your Body by God does not need your help to thrive and survive in this world. How can you help something you did not create and cannot begin to understand? *God needs no help nor interference.* This book, your Owner's Manual, will help you to figure out how to stop interfering.

God needs no help, just no interference.

If you place one artificial substance inside the BBG or do one thing to disturb it's function, then simultaneously you get hundreds of thousands of counteractions or side effects. However, when left alone, without *interference,* the BBG always knows precisely what to do to keep or get itself well, *without* side effects, and all the instructions come inside the packaging.

You hear of saving the ozone, restoring the rain forests, rescuing endangered species, and preserving our water supply. Yet, again, how can we save something we have no idea how to create? *God does not need our help to save the things He has so magnificently created, He just needs us to stop interfering.*

If we got rid of the ozone, the rain forests, all the clean water, and all the animals, we humans would *die.* However, if we got rid of the humans, the ozone, the rain forests, the clean water, and the animals would *flourish.*

When it comes to proper operation of the BBG, everyone knows that stress, lack of exercise, and eating a donut instead of an apple are bad for you. Yet war, depression, couch potatoes, and candy bars are flourishing. We keep interfering with how God created us to live and to function. As a result, many of us now live with or are even born with suffering.

Parts 2 through 5 of your Owner's Manual cover how to fuel, move, and manage stress and time with your Body by God. All guidelines follow science, technology, and, most important, the wisdom of God. This leads you away from interfering with God and toward working with Him. For optimal function, peace, success, and to extend the life of your Body by God, it is imperative that you be inspired to read, understand, and apply the guidelines.

There are laws by which the Body by God is governed. No matter how good a person you are or how noble your intentions, if you break those laws, you interfere with God. Sooner or later, if you interfere with God, you will suffer less than pleasing consequences.

The more you understand your Body by God, the more you work with God and not against Him. This allows you to better establish God's will in your life and your BBG. Using the materials in this book, myself, my family, and people all over the world are attaining higher levels of health, appearance, peace, and success than they ever imagined possible.

GOD'S RESOURCES

The wisdom for taking care of your BBG and your life can come only from God. Following and worshiping Plato, Socrates, teachers, doctors, psychiatrists, and fitness and weight-loss authors will never truly work out. If you get on your knees and call to them, they will not answer, and if you give them a bucket of dirt and some water they cannot make a human being.

Many years ago, in order to create *Body by God* and know that it was what God wanted and not just what Dr. Ben wanted, I had to rely on the following sources:

Natural Occurrence: All the methods in this book abide by the laws of nature. When applying them, you will find that they feel natural and are not overly difficult or painful. Additionally, the *Owner's Manual* programs have been successfully used by tens of thousands of BBG's in clinical and nonclinical settings all around the world.

Scientific Data: Anything that comes from God makes scientific sense. The rules of bodily function and all the laws of the universe come from God. God is the Creator of all anatomy, physiology, embryology, physics, and biochemistry. Therefore, studying and researching how the human body responds to exercise, nutrition, and anxiety helped me to better understand how God designed the BBG to eat and move and why we need to reduce stress.

Common Sense: By continuously attempting to comprehend the Bible, interpret nature, and study science, I have been able to use some common sense to tell how God has created the BBG to work and interact.

The Bible: The Bible is the best "Owner's Manual" ever created for matters of spiritual conduct, morality, and respecting God. *Body by God: The Owner's Manual for Maximized Living* is a supplement to the Bible. The Bible was my resource for developing the principles of behavior that I have recommended. Additionally, this book is a guide in the areas of nutrition, exercise, stress management, time management, and total life prosperity.

2 | THE POOR GENETICS SYNDROME (PGS) MYTH

I was born in 1966 B.A.C. (Before Anyone Cared—about exercise, diet, stress, or time management). At that time, not much lifestyle information (or even data on dental hygiene) was readily available. There weren't any popular fad diets, quick weight-loss schemes, fat-free products, sermons on tape, 7-minute ab workouts, self-empowerment books, or *Buns of Steel* videos. (Our family preferred "buns" of cinnamon.) This was a problem for my relatives, who suffered from Poor Genetics Syndrome, or PGS.

Nearly everyone I was related to who was over the age of thirty was in a constant tug-of-war battle with their weight, cholesterol levels, blood pressure, and emotions. (And anyone over age fifty put their teeth in a jar at night!)

Due to a lack of help and information, none of them could get their lives, or their bodies, under control. They thought the only way they could lose weight or eat healthier was to cut out all the foods they actually enjoyed, like pizza and ice cream, and add foods they didn't enjoy, like lettuce and celery. They also believed that only body-builders like Mr. Universe exercised, only people who took sedatives or were born into rich families were stress-free, and only religious fanatics and boring people from small farms in the Midwest prayed.

I spent the majority of my life watching the various adult members of my family painfully struggle with both their bodies and their stress levels. Many of them, including my father, died well before their time.

I was told throughout my youth that due to my genes, I could expect the same bleak outcome as my relatives before me. Rather than be discouraged, I vowed to overcome my PGS. I committed to never looking down and seeing my stomach instead of my feet, allowing my cholesterol to exceed the number of days in a year, or getting stressed over lost keys or traffic jams. I had to choose a road completely different from the road my family had chosen.

A road I now know everyone can follow.

TENDENCIES CAN BE OVERCOME

I watched my father die at only fifty-two and my mother have a stroke shortly afterward. Like other similar cases I have witnessed, my parents' poor health was not the result of a single problem—that they simply needed to eat better, exercise more, be less stressed, or better manage their time. They needed to incorporate all these things into their lifestyle. That is why this book encompasses all areas of life.

Another, and probably my greatest, gene issue was that God was not a very big part of my life growing up. In fact, His name was never said in my house unless it was in vain. I have discovered, through self-trial, clinical experience, and scientific discovery, the only way to maintain sanity and commit to a peaceful, healthy lifestyle is through God. By putting nutrition, exercise, and stress and time management together with the wisdom and love of God, I put all of the necessary pieces of the puzzle together to create wholeness, which is the basis of this book.

> **Healthy, happy people are not born, they are made . . . thank God!**

I also discovered that PGS is a myth. It doesn't even exist.

By following the rules of *Body by God: The Owner's Manual for Maximized Living,* I suffer from none of the maladies my father or my father's father suffered from at my age.

We all have some genetic tendencies to be high-strung, low-strung, headstrong, stomach-big, or heart-weak. However, these are just tendencies; they are not death sentences. Tendencies can be overcome.

TRIAL AND ERROR

I was born with the typical biological tendency to do nothing right. For me, life was one mistake, one hurt, and one catastrophe after another. It is almost embarrassing to reflect on my past. It seemed it was all rapid-fire error for me. My world was a blur of junk food, procrastination, disobedience, insubordination, illness, and injury. I don't think I was able to go an hour, never mind an entire *day*, without inflicting pain on myself or someone around me.

As a species, we are born to stray from God. No one ever had to teach me how to break windows, talk back to the teacher, lie to my parents, trash my room, cheat my friends at Go Fish, or light the backyard on fire. It all came naturally. However, I had to be *taught* every good thing. I had to be taught integrity, fairness, honesty, forgiveness, cleanliness, hard work, and every other thing that makes us decent human beings.

Look what happens when someone becomes a teenager: From the age of thirteen to age nineteen, teenagers tend to do almost everything they can to hurt themselves, destroy their future, and drive everyone around them crazy. I no longer call this period the "puberty" or "teen" years; I call it "seven years of bad luck." The fact that I survived until age twenty-one took several acts of God and some extremely patient parents, police officers, and school administrators.

There is a major misconception that healthy, optimistic people possess some sort of natural discipline or automatic tendency toward proper lifestyle or a positive mental attitude. This is rarely true. In my case, it took years of more error than trial to actually start understanding and applying the laws of health and life presented in this book.

I still make plenty of mistakes, and I probably always will. Fortunately, over time, as I have worked to become better at living in the ways I have described in this book, the errors have become less rapid-fire. I still bomb big-time on occasion, but every year there is more time between explosions and less collateral damage.

THE KEY TO LIFE: FINDING PROSPERITY

The key to changing your life—to making a true, dynamic shift in the right direction that lasts forever—is to fully understand prosperity. If you have money but poor health, you are not prosperous. If you have health but your family is falling apart and you are broke, you are not prosperous.

Similarly, if you eat well but are stressed, exercise but have bad relationships, or manage your stress but not your health, you are also not prosperous. Eventually, the one area you are lacking in will become your undoing.

Prosperity is success in not just one, but in all of the important areas of your life. To be prosperous, you must know the rules of success.

If the circumstances in some area of your life have become uncomfortable, then you need a different set of maps or plans to take you in a new and better direction. The "Four Rules of Olympic Success" presented in the following chapter are the *best* set of maps and plans for overcoming your circumstances, achieving all you desire, and discovering all God created you to be and have.

3 | THE FOUR RULES OF
OLYMPIC SUCCESS

Making any real changes in your lifestyle may be the greatest, and the most important, challenge you will face here on earth. To truly achieve, long-term, the healthy, prosperous life you were born to live, you must learn how to succeed. The Four Rules of Olympic Success will teach you the rules of winning employed by Olympians, the people who are the masters of success.

The athletes who make the Olympic team or go on to win medals at the actual Olympics are all ridiculously, incredibly talented at winning. They are literally the best—or even better—*at success*.

If you played a sport in high school or watched one regularly, then you can probably recall someone either on your team or from another one that was so amazingly talented that he or she just dominated your town or state.

Statistically, that dominant, "best" athlete from your town or state most likely never even made a college team. That makes college athletes the "best of the best."

Then, of all of those college "best of the best" athletes, some will even be good enough to go on to try and make an Olympic team. They will then enter an Olympic trial. In an Olympic trial, the "best of the best" will often be beaten, or even beaten badly. This makes Olympians the "best of the best of the best."

Even more fascinating is that at the actual Olympics, the "best of the best of the best" will also lose or even lose *big* to an Olympic medalist. This makes an Olympic Medalist the "best of the best of the best of the best."

To be an Olympian—or even more, an Olympic gold-medal-winning champion—is so remarkable, it is almost beyond the realm of comprehension.

I wrestled in junior high, high school, and college, and I continue to coach high school and college kids in wrestling and weight lifting today. While I had dreams of being the best of the best of the best, the fact was, I had no idea how to do that. Effectively, I never achieved it. That is why I became extremely excited when I had the opportunity to treat and counsel hundreds of Olympians and dozens of Olympic medalists. While at first my excitement was about having a chance to work with champion athletes, my joy ultimately came not so much in being their doctor, but in being their *student*.

I not only had the opportunity to work with these incredible human beings and observe and participate in their training and preparation, I also was able to go to the Olympics and other world events with them. Over the years, I began to see the major differences between losers and winners at the highest level possible. The rules of success that made the best of the best of the best athletes winners are also the rules of success in life. I observed that there were Four Rules of Olympic Success.

THE FOUR RULES OF OLYMPIC SUCCESS

Following the Four Rules of Olympic Success will ensure that when you apply the principles of your *Body by God: The Owner's Manual for Maximized Living* to your life, you will have the best chance to succeed. The four rules are:

1. Discover and develop your gifts.
2. Possess a superior plan.
3. Follow the plan.
4. Be inspired to win.

Rule #1: Discover and Develop Your Gifts

Olympians all possess God-given gifts that have made them physically or technically superior to their opponents. Olympians are born with the gifts of speed, strength, and athletic ability. Yet, if these people never discover or develop these gifts, then the gifts will be wasted. They will never become Olympians.

You also possess very special and unique gifts. As a matter of fact, your gifts and talents are designed to serve God's will and enrich the lives of others. Your gifts and talents are far more important than the physical attributes of any athlete—Olympic, professional, or otherwise. But if you never eat right, exercise, get your stress under control, manage your time, or discover and practice using your gifts, you will never win either.

You've got skills. You have been given gifts, though those gifts may be hidden within you. These gifts are from God, which gives you the potential to be the "best of the best of the best of the best" and live a wonderful, healthy, gold-medal life. All you have to do is seek, develop, and not waste your gifts.

> Each one should use whatever gift he has received to serve others, faithfully administering God's grace in its various forms. (1 Pet. 4:10)

PLAY YOUR DRUM FOR HIM—
SEEK AND FULFILL YOUR DESTINY

A popular Christmas song tells of a little boy who feels that because of his worldly position and lack of money, he is unworthy and has nothing fit to give to the newborn Jesus.

Isn't that just like us? While God has given us so much, we feel that we have nothing to give back to God and others. Even though God wants, and others need, to love us and to receive love from us, we have a constant feeling of not being valuable.

Fortunately for the "Newborn King," and all the rest of us who have enjoyed that song at Christmastime, the little boy figures out that he does have a gift—a gift God has given him. He realizes any gift that comes from God is worthy to give a king. The Little Drummer Boy then proceeds not only to give his gift and play for Him, but he plays his best for Him.

You are incredibly valuable. God has given you gifts that He desires you to express to fill the world's needs. You have an obligation to realize your potential. In God's ideal scene, everybody is fully expressing their gifts in a way that serves Him and assists Him by helping the world.

When you are using your gifts to fulfill whatever mission God has given you in life, you will find yourself feeling worthy and exceedingly effective, healthy, joyful, and at peace.

Play your drum, or whatever other instrument you play, for him, and play your best. You have gifts fit for the King. Discover and develop these gifts—seek and fulfill your destiny.

No matter where you are in life—shepherd, prince, pauper, drummer boy, or drummer girl—God loves you and is counting on you. No matter what place you may have found yourself in life, God is standing by at all times, waiting for you to feel important enough to come and play your drum for Him.

HOW TO FIND AND EXPRESS YOUR GIFTS

Your gifts contain your destiny. They are made up of the things you are good at and the things you love to do. When you find and develop your gifts and "go for it," there is no situation or circumstance you cannot overcome.

My best friend, Brett, comes from a very poor part of the world. However, all of his life he has felt that God chose him for greatness. He knew that he possessed a powerful future.

Brett discovered his gifts, developed them, and his heart told him that God would one day use those gifts to bless others. This gave him the courage to seek and fulfill his destiny. As a result of his attitude and his sincere desire to dedicate his life and his gifts to God and the people around him, he is very happy and successful today. He did this despite the fact that the environment he grew up in was overwhelmingly challenging.

On the contrary, many of his family members, who are also very gifted and talented people, have never escaped their impoverished situation. They failed to use their gifts and express the greatness God placed inside them. As a result, they never had the ability or the courage to leave their circumstances, and they still suffer in a place that Brett, who played his drum for God, rose above.

> *No plan of yours [God's] can be thwarted.* (Job 42:2)

Rule #2: Possess a Superior Plan

The Olympic coaches spend hours each week watching videos of the athletes on their teams, as well as the athletes their teams will be competing against, in order to develop a plan for victory. One of my old coaches used to say, "Everyone wants to win on game day, but the one who actually wins is the one who *plans to win* on game day."

Even though Olympians possesses great and developed gifts, if they do not possess a superior plan for success, they may not end up where they want to be—on the gold-medal stand.

Many of the lifestyle plans available to us possess information that is not factual or scientific, and that comes from man's perspective only—not God's. As a result, these are not *superior* plans.

Body by God takes information that comes from reviewing the cases of thousands of people who are actually performing the plan, utilizing the latest science in understanding the body's function, and looking at life from God's perspective. The plans in this book are superior plans designed for an Olympian ability to succeed.

> **The only thing greater than the desire to win is the desire to plan to win.**

DAVID VS. GOLIATH

Goliath was over nine feet tall (and about five hundred–plus pounds). He wore a bronze helmet on his huge head and donned a coat of scale armor weighing five thousand shekels; on his legs he wore bronze greaves, and a bronze javelin was slung on his back. His spear shaft had an iron point that weighed six hundred shekels. All in all, this behemoth carried around three hundred pounds of armor and weaponry into battle, for a total weight of approximately eight hundred pounds.

Goliath was the world's first undefeated heavyweight champion. Wanting to bring victory to God's army and knowing the incredible draw a fight with the champ Goliath would bring, King Saul did everything he could to find a contender. In an effort to encourage willing opponents, Saul offered the man who killed Goliath great wealth, tax exemption, and even his daughter. That may not seem like much now, but that was a good payday back in Bible times.

Although David was only a lightweight, he was chosen by God as the number one contender to take on the heavyweight champ. While this match took place way before cable or pay-per-view existed, the Bible does a good job of covering the bout.

The line on the fight had David as a 100:1 underdog. But what the line did not know was that God does not choose underdogs. If God picks you, you are the overwhelming favorite to win.

God chose the man with the superior plan. Earlier previews of David's life show that when David was tending his father's flocks and a lion or a bear would get a sheep, he would strike the predator and take the sheep out of its mouth. If the beast turned on him, he grabbed it by the hair and killed it. That is a man with a plan. While Goliath's war plan was to use the same tactics he had always used to defeat mere men, David's plan was to use the same tactics, skills, and methods he had used to defeat vicious, wild animals.

As a result of his superior planning, David the lightweight knocked out the heavyweight Goliath in the first round. With one punch (rock).

Following his big win, David continued to go through trials and tribulations brought on him by his enemies—and even by his own mistakes. While most people would allow this kind of stress to crush them, David used these challenges to plan for the more important tasks that lay ahead. God knew David would endure and plan. That is why He chose a sheepherder from among all the warriors and princes of Israel to be king.

You have your own Goliaths to fight. You become the overwhelming favorite to win if you follow Rule #2 and possess a superior plan to defeat them.

Rule #3: Follow the Plan

In preparation for Olympic and world competitions, U.S. athletes attend training camps several months before the event. These training camps involve leaving friends and family behind to go live at an Olympic training center, either in America or somewhere near the site of the competition. Most of the world's training centers are in small, out-of-the-way towns, and the accommodations are quite a bit below "five-star."

After a difficult night's sleep on rough, dormitory-style beds, a shower with no hot water, and a meal that often contained several mystery foods that were far from being ideal for training, the athletes endure two to three rigorous practices a day. These practices include whatever it takes to follow the superior plan that has been developed by coaches and advisors. At the end of these difficult camps, if the athletes have done as they've been told, they will be ready for victory.

Unfortunately, while teams of this caliber always have a superior plan, sometimes the athletes do not follow the plan. Injuries, procrastination, laziness, or burnout often will deter some of the athletes from adhering to the schedule and create failure to succeed in the competition.

The pages of this book contain the plan—the information necessary for you to be victorious in all areas of health and life. However, the success you will experience can be measured only by how well you learn and apply the knowledge obtained from your Owner's Manual.

Knowledge = Results

KNOWING WITHOUT DOING IS NOT KNOWING

In Hosea 4:6, God says, "My people are destroyed from lack of knowledge." God doesn't say, "My people are destroyed for lack of Bibles, health books, audiotapes, videos, motivational speakers, or Web sites." That is because there is now, and has always been, more than enough information; it's just that there has never been enough *knowledge*.

The word for "knowledge" in the verse quoted above also means "understanding" and/or "wisdom." Understanding and wisdom do not mean that you only come across information, but that you also *act on it*. In the Bible, *"knowledge"* denotes action or the ability to perform what knowledge claims is true.

While there are a lot of sources of information and plans for leading a better life, people continue to be destroyed because of a "lack of knowledge." This is because there is a big difference between information and real biblical knowledge. Information is *knowing;* and real biblical knowledge is *doing*.

Knowing without doing is not knowing. If you truly "know" something, it means you are doing it. As a product of that equation, knowledge = results.

In 1998, I went to Sweden with the U.S. World Greco Roman Wrestling Team to help them get ready to compete for the World Championships. Part of my interest in going was not only to work with the athletes, but also to study the Swedish people and their lifestyle. At that time, Sweden had less than half the amount of heart disease and cancer as the U.S. and only a fraction of the amount of infant deaths.

I was not there very long before I discovered many subtle differences in their way of living that would account for their superior health. However, the biggest reason for their better-functioning, longer-lasting Bodies by God was not so much what they ate for breakfast, how much they exercised, or how they managed their stress as it was *why* they lived this way.

When I was taking a cab ride from the airport, I noticed there were an incredible number of McDonald's restaurants along the road. In certain areas there were even McDonald's right across the street from each other. I eventually made a comment to the cabdriver about how surprised I was to see so many fast-food chains in a healthy country like Sweden. He then gave me a lecture on Scandinavian living that changed my perception of health forever.

He told me that when the first McDonald's arrived, the Swedish people actually shut it down. They did this simply by refusing to eat there. He said no one would eat their food because they *knew* it was unhealthy. The Swedes would not purchase food from this McDonald's until they agreed to lower the amount of fat in their sauces and reduce the amount of grease they used when cooking the food. Even since the restaurants complied, the driver said, the people still *know* to go there only on rare occasions and they *know* not to order too much.

The real reason Sweden, as well as most other countries in the world, is healthier than the U.S. is that if the people there know something, they *act* accordingly. If the people of Sweden have knowledge, or the right plan for doing things that are good for them, they follow that plan, which makes their knowledge real biblical knowledge. The result is healthier adults and children.

Americans know that fast-food restaurants are unhealthy, yet we line up at their doors every day.

In America, knowledge has exceeded action. We have a plan, but many people do not follow the plan. This makes our knowledge only useless information. The result is, as Hosea 4:6 says, God's people are being destroyed.

> Commit to the LORD whatever you do, and your plans will succeed. (Prov. 16:3)

Rule #4: Be Inspired to Win

Great Olympians are more than motivated to win; they are inspired to be victorious. Motivation itself is often weak and temporary. It comes purely from a short term desire to win some sort of material prize such as a medal, a trophy, or money. Inspiration, however, comes from an inner, burning passion to do things for God, country, or a cause that burns deep within the heart. While many people throughout history have won through sheer giftedness or planning, the greatest were those who were *inspired*.

MOTIVATION VS. INSPIRATION

Motivation is driven by earthly desire and a need to gain self-satisfaction;
Inspiration is driven by heavenly success and a desire to please God.

Motivation is like showering or brushing your teeth—you need to do it every day;
Inspiration happens once and is there forever.

Motivation can be broken;
Inspiration can be blocked but never truly goes away.

Motivation ends during tough or inconvenient times;
Inspiration endures hardship and failure.

Motivation yields to excuses;
Inspiration will not stop until it sees results.

Motivation is like tiptoeing into a cold pool;
Inspiration gives you the courage to dive right in, take the leap, and go for it.

Motivation changes with changing emotions;
Inspiration is stronger than a particular feeling at a particular moment.

Motivation takes no effort or focus;
Inspiration takes the effort of focusing on God and the responsibilities we all have.

Motivation creates the discipline and interest to change temporarily;
Inspiration creates the obedience to change permanently.

Motivation is driven by a love for self;
Inspiration is driven by a love for God.

No one can follow a plan for long by sheer force of will alone. Without inspiration, when people step onto the court, the mat, or the field of play, they are so overwhelmed or afraid of losing that they do not do what it takes to win. In the end, they create the very thing they feared—a loss. They will not have allowed themselves to win. If David were not inspired, he would have been so afraid of Goliath that when he threw the rock he would have been lucky to hit him on the elbow.

Inspiration is the greatest reason for success, and lack of it is the greatest reason for failure. When your mission is clear and you have not lost sight of your goal, it is not too difficult to stay motivated to follow your plan or apply your knowledge. Unfortunately, all too often, as the cares of the world and the challenges of life arise, missions get cloudy, motivation dims, and it is easy to lose focus on goals. At these times, most plans are interfered with, and the courage to strive for victory becomes less than a distant memory.

Once you get the big picture, inspiration rarely fades totally from sight. You may rest at times, but you will never quit.

While the Olympics are an extremely important event, your daily events are even more important. Throwing a ball, swimming, running down a track, or rolling around on a mat in tights by yourself or with another person is not as important as your real job, your family obligations, your spiritual responsibilities, and your own happiness and longevity.

You are the "real Olympian."

Get inspired! Every time you win, you may not get a medal on earth as you would if you could outrun or jump higher than someone else, but God pins one up for you in heaven. Shakespeare, Lincoln, Ruth (from the Bible—not Babe), Jeremiah, Isaiah, Peter, John, and Paul (the apostles not the Beatles) never won a basketball game, kicked a field goal, or got a score of 10 on the balance beam, but their names are cherished and will be remembered for all eternity.

Inspiration is the father of obedience.

YOU ARE A WORK IN PROGRESS

The Bible is one of the primary resources I used to write and support the science and beliefs of *Body by God*. I chose the Bible not only because it is the Word of God, but also because many of the people and principles discussed in the Bible have shaped history and mirror the kinds of lives God desires for us all.

When you learn about the men and women God speaks of in the Bible, you cannot help but be inspired by their amazing ability to overcome their own humanness. They overcame their cravings, feelings, and emotions in a manner that caused God to bless them and reveal Himself to them in countless pleasurable ways. Many of them also managed to get an incredible amount done in a very short period of time. (Jesus' ministry lasted only three years!)

These heroes made choices in regard to their bodies and their actions that appear so disciplined and faithful it almost goes beyond what we would consider possible today. They are definitely great individuals to model and learn from.

People like Joseph and Daniel had what seemed to be an uncanny ability to control their emotions and stay focused on a purpose despite hideous circumstances.

When you read about the accomplishments of men like David and Paul, you have to be curious as to how it was possible to accomplish so much in so many areas of the world in just one lifetime.

When you look at Moses and Jesus, one of the many things you end up desiring is to find yourself in a place similar to theirs where you are actually hearing God's voice directing you toward your destiny and reaching out to millions.

I have to assume that during the first two to three thousand years of our existence, there were probably more than just the few dozen heroes God talks about in the Bible. I would venture to say there were probably people who did things even greater than those mentioned in the text. What makes the Bible such an incredible tool of self-discovery and success is not so much what the people achieved, but why they achieved. They did not accomplish things for their own fame or fortune. The great people of the Bible did not accomplish things for their own good. They accomplished things for the good of God.

INSPIRED OBEDIENCE

People think I have discipline. In one instance, a person introducing me onstage to speak at a seminar stated as part of the introduction, "Dr. Ben is the most disciplined guy I know." However, the truth is, I do not have discipline. Just ask my wife. I am terrible about putting my shoes back in the closet, rinsing out my oatmeal bowl, and filling up the car with gas.

What Moses, Joseph, Daniel, David, Jesus, Paul, and I—to a much lesser degree—have is not discipline; it is obedience. Obedience is a sincere desire to do that which pleases God and supports His work here on earth and beyond. While discipline is self-motivated, *obedience is inspired*. Obedience is inspired by a love for God.

People do not respond to "have to" or "should." For instance, "Billy, you *have to* clean your room," or "I really *should* not eat dessert." "Have to" and "should" require discipline. Discipline is like motivation; ultimately, it runs short. Motivation and discipline are "for me." The reason obedience is much more powerful and effective is because obedience is not "for me"; it is "for God." Inspiration comes through the love one has for God. That is what makes inspiration *the father of obedience.*

Regular people normally fail at the things they have made commitments to, such as diets, exercise, and marriages, because they have committed to these things for themselves. These types of commitments require discipline.

On the other hand, Bible heroes did not fail at their commitments because they were committing for the Lord. They loved God so much that they did not require discipline. They were inspired to be obedient. As Proverbs 16:3 says, "Commit to the LORD whatever you do, and your plans will succeed."

When it comes to levels of stress, body weight, relationships, finances, or fitness levels, you did not just end up with them; you created them.

If you are having problems in any or all of these areas, you may have identified the problem as a lack of discipline. I would like you to change that phrase from "a lack of discipline" (for me) to "a lack of inspiration and obedience" (for God). Psalm 24:1 says, "The earth is the LORD's, and everything in it, the world, and all who live in it." You, your body, your life, and the entire world you live in are not your own. They are God's. By committing all of these things and your entire future to Him, you will be inspired to discover the obedience necessary to do as Proverbs 16:3 says and "succeed."

The important thing to remember is that most of the really cool Bible heroes got off to some pretty slow starts. Some of them had pretty bad middles as well. This is great news because if you are like me, you not only have gotten off to some bad starts, you have also had some rough middles. Fortunately, the most important part of a race is not the beginning or the middle . . . it is the finish.

Just think of yourself as a construction zone. You are a "work in progress." While your body and your life may look as if they have just been hit by a wrecking ball, remember that for a beautiful new building to be erected, sometimes the old, worn-out structure that was standing there has to be destroyed. For the beautiful, new butterfly to be born and soar to another level, the old, ugly caterpillar has to die.

In reality, there really are no caterpillars, only inspired butterflies that love God so much that they are willing to show obedience to being a "work in progress."

THE BODY BY GOD 40-DAY PLANS

You are a work in progress. Going from caterpillar to butterfly is a process . . . a slow process. However, during the course of this process there is constant improvement. There is a slow and steady progression toward being all that God created the caterpillar to be.

That is why I created the Body by God 40-Day Plan. In this plan, the goal is to get 1 percent better for God each day for a period of forty days. Anyone can do that! In fact, the programs in this book are so simple and easy to follow that most people continue to get 1 percent better each day for the rest of their lives.

See the Body by God 40-Day Plan in the "Life by God" section at the end of your *Owner's Manual for Maximized Living*. It will totally revolutionize your entire life in only forty days!

The Body by God *Overnight Success* 40-Day Plans

(Alternative 40-Day Body by God Plans)

Deliberate and continual change is God's way. Nonetheless, if you want miraculous changes, overnight, follow the Body by God 40-Day Overnight Success Programs. These plans for nutrition or exercise will get quicker, more dramatic changes in your health and appearance and help you become a star of before-and-after photos. Follow them both together and you will become an "overnight success."

While stress management and time management improve with learning over time, it is possible with nutrition and exercise to see results literally overnight.

PART TWO | FUELING YOUR BODY BY GOD

4 | FOOD BY GOD: THE "UN-DIET"

Nutritional decisions are important not only to you; they are obviously impor-tant to God. Right from the start, food has had a huge role in establishing our relationships with Him. Look at Adam and Eve: A bad neighbor convinces Adam and Eve to cheat on their diet, and the next thing you know, instead of eating grapes and frolicking naked in the Garden of Eden, Adam is wolfing down a jelly donut and a cup of coffee in rush-hour traffic at six in the morning, while Eve is feeding the kids a bowl of Froot Loops with milk from a cow before dropping them off at day care.

One bad meal started this whole crazy game. But it should come as no surprise: Throughout history, not only our health but our relationships with God have often been developed and tested through our need to eat.

When Moses marched thousands through the desert, he was continually confronted with challenges. While the absence of air-conditioning and a lack of comfortable sandals were obviously huge obstacles, it was a shortage of food and beverages the Bible chooses to focus on. Because there was no take-out food or convenience stores back then, when hunger and thirst brought Moses to his knees he was forced to turn to God. When he did, his prayers were answered. In fact, it was then God invented the very first free home-delivery service by sending bread down from heaven at no charge—conveniently right to their front tent door—to show how much He blesses and loves those who seek Him. Later, He even supplied a rock water fountain!

Throughout history, the mystery of nutrition has caused most everyone to slip up or suffer. Fortunately, the advantage of suffering is that it usually brings about a desire to seek God. And this is probably why at some point throughout the year, nearly every religion and culture focuses on some sort of eating ritual.

Since the literal beginning of time, the natural temptation of food has been so great, it has been one of the main themes of the Bible and continues to be a part of many stories of today. In this section of your Owner's Manual, I will unlock the historic food mystery of the ages and show you how to easily and painlessly put this age-old problem of food to rest.

THE UN-DIET: HOW GOD WANTS YOU TO EAT

For centuries, there has been a tremendous amount of diet and nutritional information available. However, it obviously has not worked. American people are now more over-weight than ever, and nutritionally related diseases are at an all-time high and beginning to spread abroad.

The guidelines for fueling your Body by God that you will read in this part are not about a diet, because it is clear that diets are too hard and painful and thus do not work. Instead, we will focus on the "Un-Diet."

Following are some popular myths about dieting countered by Un-Diet truths.

DIET MYTHS V. UN-DIET TRUTHS

Diet Myth #1: Diet = Deprivation.

Un-Diet Truth: The Un-Diet is not about eating only bland, tasteless foods, restricting portions, or cutting calories. In fact, while the Un-Diet does recommend certain foods, if you follow the "Un-Diet Food Guide" found on pages 82–84, you do not have to change the foods you eat at all.

Diet Myth #2: Eat like an elephant, look like an elephant.

Un-Diet Truth: If you are eating the foods God intended you to eat and/or eating the way He intended you to eat (following the Un-Diet Food Guide), you will *never* look like an elephant.

Diet Myth #3: If you crave, you cave (once you cheat or go off your diet, it's over).

Un-Diet Truth: Taking short vacations from proper eating is part of the Un-Diet. Eating a food you crave is actually part of the plan.

Diet Myth #4: You can trick the body into thinness and better health.

Un-Diet Truth: God's body cannot be tricked; it must be looked on in awe. Diets that restrict foods or use only one kind of food category, such as a protein-only diet, may trick the body into change in the short term. However, they *never* work in the long term. Eliminating an entire food group cannot be healthy because God would not have placed those foods on the face of the earth in the first place if they were not to be eaten.

The Un-Diet uses a balance of foods *including* fruits, vegetables, whole grains like oats and basmati rice, as well as protein, all eaten at the right time to create real, lasting health and thinness.

Diet Myth #5: It's best to get a balance of protein, fats, and carbohydrates at every meal.

Un-Diet Truth: Varying amounts of carbohydrates, proteins, and fats are needed at different *times* throughout the day. Additionally, the Body by God does not digest protein and carbohydrates the same way so they should not be consumed in large amounts together.

Diet Myth #6: There is a cookie-cutter diet that works for all people or all people with certain backgrounds or body types.

Un-Diet Truth: God made people like snowflakes; no two are exactly alike.

Diet Myth #7: "Low-," "reduced-," "-free," "no-" foods are "health and diet foods," and food that is good for you is expensive.

Un-Diet Truth: Synthetic, refined, or chemically altered foods that say: "low-fat," "reduced-cholesterol," "lactose-free," "no-sugar," etc., will never grant long-term health or thinness. Anything man creates for the BBG to eat cannot be considered "health and diet food." Additionally, these foods *are* expensive. Food by God is the only health and diet food there is, and overall it costs a lot less.

Owner's Manual Truth Tip:
Life is not a game of perfect.

Improving how you fuel your Body by God shows respect for the body God has given you. This should not produce frustration or make you feel pressured to eat well. It should, however, make you feel inspired to do "better." God knows you are not perfect and will never be. Life is not a game of perfection.

I have worked with professional and Olympic teams and athletes of all kinds. Whether their sport is golf, basketball, wrestling, tennis, or baseball, one thing they all have in common is that they can make a mistake—in fact, several mistakes—and still win their game or match. An individual or a team can miss shots, experience turnovers, commit errors, or slice a couple of shots into the woods and—despite their mistakes—still become champions.

Improving any habit, particularly your eating habits, is extremely difficult. This commonly leads to making mistakes. But do not let that stop you from getting in the game.

DIETING IS NOT A GAME OF PERFECT EITHER

You are not looking for the perfect diet. Rarely does anyone eat perfectly for even one day, never mind a whole week or a whole lifetime! The important part is to get started. Just get in the game because life can only improve if you get off the bench. You are never going to follow a diet without error—and you don't have to. When you make your mistakes, get back in the game, and remember, you can make several errors and still win. You lose only if you lose hope.

> We know that suffering produces perseverance; perseverance, character; and character, hope. And hope does not disappoint us. (Rom. 5:3–5)

EATING FOR THREE

In this world, committing to doing anything right is difficult. No matter what you do, there will always be challenges and natural temptations that pull you away from doing good. I have found that when I am doing something purely for my own sake, it is significantly more difficult to stay committed than if I am doing it for others.

Because a healthier eating program gives you more energy, greater strength, increased mental awareness, and significantly increases the time you will spend here on the planet, what you put in your mouth affects others. When you consider what you are going to put in your mouth (which most people do not consider at all), remember that if you lead a better, longer life, you can do a tremendous amount more for God and the people you love. Pregnant women always say that they are eating for two. I always say that I am eating for three:

1. for me
2. for the people around me
3. for God

When I remind myself of that, I am far more likely to put the right things in my mouth.

DANIEL ATE FOR THREE

In the book of Daniel, the king ordered his chief court official to bring him young men who were without any physical defect, handsome, showed aptitude for every kind of learning, were well-informed, and were qualified to serve in the king's palace. One of these young men was Daniel.

The king apportioned to these men a daily amount of food and wine from his table. This royal food was unhealthy and made up of things that had been sacrificed to other gods. Despite incredible pressure from the king, temptation from his own body, and the fact that every one around him was eating this way, Daniel chose to be faithful to the Lord and resolved not to defile his body with the royal food.

Daniel asked the king's chief court official for permission not to eat this food. God, seeing Daniel's respect for Him and his own body, caused the official to show favor and sympathy for Daniel. So while the official was concerned that he would get in trouble for letting Daniel look worse than the other men, who were still eating the royal food, he was willing to grant Daniel's request.

Daniel convinced the official to feed him only vegetables and water for ten days and then test him against the other men. At the end of this small research project, Daniel looked healthier and better nourished than any of the other men. As a result, the guard allowed Daniel to stick to God's nutrition plan instead of the king's.

Daniel's courage and obedience, which came through a love for God, brought him many blessings. God blessed Daniel with knowledge, understanding of all kinds of literature, and learning that was ten times greater than that of anyone else in the whole kingdom. Later, God saved Daniel from the evil of men and the mouths of lions. He also gave Daniel the ability to see and interpret visions and dreams that eventually would change the course of history.

In this world, to the faithful go the blessings. Daniel knew he was eating for three. Because he followed God's nutritional plan, he not only received blessings far beyond what he could have imagined, he also ended up blessing God and everyone else around him.

God is looking to work with you. Eating poorly makes that difficult to do. When you eat poorly it is not that you are cursed, it is just that you are not blessed. However, when eating for three, what you will ultimately find is not painful sacrifice, but pleasures that far exceed any of those foods that might have tempted you.

As it is written in the Bible and as you have experienced in your own life, what you are eating affects not only you, but God and everyone around you. To be blessed like Daniel, anytime you begin to eat, say, "I am eating for three."

IF LIFE WERE LIKE A BOX OF CHOCOLATES . . .

My entire family comes from New York City. It is the birthplace of the jelly donut, the cheesecake, and the knish; and it is where pizza and the "street hot dog" were perfected. As a result of our origin, food always was and still is a major part of my family's life. That is why when I was growing up, nearly everyone in my family and most of our family's friends had a weight problem.

So standard was this whole weight issue in my genetic line that at a very young age I was told I, too, would one day be fat. At an age when other kids were being told they would one day become the president of the United States, a famous actor, or that they would discover a cure for cancer, it was being prophesied to me that I soon would have big pants.

Being told that very long belts and the need to shop for clothes in special stores were in my future, I became extremely concerned. The problem was, I wasn't exactly sure what to do. Eating a lot of whatever tasted best was all I had ever known.

I was raised on the three C's: Cow products, Chemicals, and empty Calories. My two favorite meals were Fruity Pebbles and pepperoni pizza. Furthermore, if it wasn't full of sugar and colorings, I wouldn't drink it.

Looking back, I can see that my eating habits were not doing much for my health. Like most American kids, I spent more time in doctors' offices than I did on the playground. I had ear problems, allergies, chronic upper-respiratory infections, growing pains, and had several different organs of immunity (tonsils and adenoids) removed. In fact, in every picture I have of my childhood, my nose was running. (A wet nose may mean a dog is well, but not a child.)

If I wasn't in the doctor's office, I was in the principal's office. In today's American society, they would have had me on a Ritalin IV drip. Luckily, back then they used writing sentences and erasing chalkboards as a form of discipline instead of psychotropic drugs.

Unfortunately, although I was continuously ill, my nose was always running, and I constantly struggled to sit quietly in a classroom, no one ever even considered the possibility that my problems may have been related to all the sugar, dairy products, caffeine, and food coloring coursing through my veins.

LIVING TO EAT OR EATING TO LIVE?

My first nutritional insight came from my eighth-grade health teacher. To this day, I can remember hearing him say, "Some people eat to live, and some people live to eat." I thought, *That's me! That's my problem! I live to eat!*

Before he said that, I didn't even know food was necessary for survival. I just thought we ate because we liked food. Unfortunately, without the knowledge or resources to change my diet, the way I ate did not change much throughout my youth. As a result, pains, symptoms, as well as a nasty disposition all affected me on a regular basis my entire childhood.

By the grace of God, my internal organs somehow managed to survive long enough to go to college. By then the joint problems, blood-sugar issues, allergies, and colds that had plagued me all my life were worse than ever. My first year, I considered 8:00 A.M. classes cruel and barbaric. In order to survive as a freshman, I had to figure out a way to schedule all my classes in the afternoons.

I chose a college with a good wrestling program in hopes of improving on my injury-hampered high-school career. But my health was so bad, I was not able to compete in wrestling my first year. The back, knee, and shoulder problems I struggled with in high school were continuing to plague me. I spent more time with college trainers and local orthopedists than I ever did in the college practice room.

Frustrated, I decided to ask one of the assistant wrestling coaches if there was anything I could do. He told me that if I was ever going to be a great wrestler, I would have to change what I was eating. My first thought was, *What does eating have to do with my health, my joints, and my wrestling?* I knew eating affected weight, but how could food affect my shoulders, back, knees, and immune system?

Willing to try anything, I began to work on passing the familiar sugared cereal and dessert lines in the cafeteria and instead stopping at the foreign fruit and salad sections. While Fruity Pebbles, pizza, and water with sugar and coloring continued to be high on my priority list, I eventually started to exchange the three C's for some better choices.

I gradually began to see changes in my health, my joints, and the look and performance of my body. In my second year of college, I was able to take morning classes, didn't have one cold all year, and I became an Academic All-American in wrestling.

I became so interested in nutrition that I decided to get a degree in it. As my knowledge of health and nutrition grew, it began to occur to me that eating not only had a tremendous amount to do with why my wrestling suffered, it was also a big part of the reason my relatives were dying young. I realized that gaining control of what I was eating would not only help me win matches, it would help me gain control of my destiny.

Living to eat is something a lot of us are caught up in. In fact, I am not sure I will ever fully recover from the "live to eat" psychology. While many people wake up and consider what they are going to do for the day, I still oftentimes wake up and think less about what I am going to do during the day and more about what I am going to eat during the day. Just as I started doing in college, the trick has been not to give up loving to eat, but to get better at choosing what I eat.

Again, good nutrition does not mean perfect eating. By comprehending even some of the guidelines for fueling your BBG and getting better and better about applying them, you, too, will look better, win more matches, have a much drier nose, and receive many more blessings.

There are no failures, only opportunities to learn.

MAKING CHANGE EASY

If you continue to look at nutrition the way most people do—"I'm on a diet" or "I'm off a diet"—you'll never learn. You are bound to a life of yo-yo eating where your weight, your health, and your peace of mind go up and down forever.

The key to the future is to learn from the past as well as the present. The bottom line is, when you first attempt to improve your eating, you are still going to like pizza, candy, and ice cream. To create a way of eating that will cause stable, predictable results, you cannot believe that you "caved because you craved." Rather than believing you have failed every time you eat something you feel you shouldn't have, learn from the experience. Then, the next time you are in the same situation, you can look at how you felt in the past when you ate the wrong thing and thus begin to do better in the present.

The other extremely important thing to remember is that any long-term, healthy eating plan includes meals or days that are made up of the things you love. Never say never. Never say to yourself, "That is it. That is the last piece of chocolate I will ever eat." First of all, you will instantly want it because you can't have it. Second, as you will see, well-placed vacations from the program are an important part of the Un-Diet. Sometimes you need a break. Like any vacation, these breaks are necessary for mental and emotional health and to enjoy life to its fullest. In that way, a well-placed piece of chocolate every once in a while is actually good for you.

When I used to try dieting, the decision to eat oatmeal for breakfast instead of

Sugar Smacks, or tuna and a baked potato for lunch instead of a cheeseburger and fries, was painful. The pain was also cumulative. The longer I dieted, the more powerful the desire to binge was and the longer it would last. Just realize, you are not psychotic if you have gotten up in the middle of the night and eaten a whole bag of cookies or a whole tub of ice cream as a result of the dieting process. I have been there. (I thank God every week for the Un-Diet Vacation Food Program.)

In my family, when we used to say the diet starts Monday, we would gain more weight on Sunday than we would ever lose on the diet.

What has been neat and totally subconscious is that over the years, I have gotten to the point where ninety-nine times out of one hundred, I prefer the oatmeal and the tuna to the junk-food alternatives that do not allow me to look or feel my best. I even prefer the cleaner, fresher, less oily taste of healthy meals now.

What I eventually discovered was that all the permanent pleasures associated with eating well—such as better health, higher energy, more restful sleep, looking your best, increased libido, improved work performance, and a happier frame of mind—usually far outweigh the temporary pleasures of the taste. When this is not the case, I eat something I crave, and then I move on. Sometimes I get off the plan for a few days, but all the pleasurable things about eating well start to go away and I feel sick. Then I look forward to getting back to what are now my new eating habits.

HOW TO GAIN EIGHT POUNDS IN FOURTEEN DAYS

When I first got out of college, I began to work in various clinics and gyms as a nutritionist and weight-loss counselor. My first patient was a woman whom a friend of mine was dating. She was beginning to put on a lot of weight, and she wanted to get it under control. (My friend wanted her to get it under control as well.)

As I had not created the Un-Diet yet, I gave her the standard diet program recommended by the nutritional science world at the time. It consisted of following a point scale. Each carbohydrate, protein, and fat gram was worth a certain number of points, and you were allowed only so many points per meal and per day. The object of this point system was to make sure you got the nutrients you needed while taking in only a certain amount of calories. One obvious problem with this method was that if you ate a cookie, that was it for food for the day.

Despite the fact that she handed in a diet diary every week showing that she was abiding by the system, every time she came in to see me, she had gained weight. At the end of her second week, she had gained eight pounds.

About that time, my friend called me and began to question what I was doing. In fact, he said, "You obviously have no idea what you are doing!"

With the painful reality that his girlfriend was packing on pounds at an alarming rate while under my care, and that the other clients I had started on the program also were gaining weight, I began to wonder if maybe he wasn't right.

The next day, as I pulled into the weight-loss clinic parking lot, I noticed my friend's girlfriend had arrived before me. I pulled up right next to her car to park, and as I got out of my car, I couldn't help but notice that her passenger seat was covered with colored sprinkles. As it turns out, part of her nutritionist appointment included a trip to Dairy Queen (a snack that had not managed to make its way onto the weekly diet diary). I thought to myself, *Great job. As a result of your care, she now not only has an eating disorder, she's a compulsive liar!*

My schooling and my own attitudes about the need to eat well had made me into the "Food Nazi." In the early part of my career, I had reached a point where I believed anyone who did not eat right was just wrong. Subconsciously, I may even have believed that heaven had a weight limit. I was so bad that when it was time for the lunch break at a seminar I was attending, the speaker actually said, "I do not recommend you eat with Dr. Ben, he'll make you afraid of your food."

After years of watching all my weight-loss patients gain an average of four pounds a week, and having all my diabetes patients end up needing to double their insulin, I finally changed my attitude and my method.

My attitude changed from one of law to one of love. My desire to help people had made me too harsh and legalistic. I realized that God does not love you any less if you do not eat well. And neither do I. We may have difficulty helping you, but we love you just the same.

I now have a system, which works for everyone. It helps you to improve nutritional habits, create better health, and to find your ideal weight. If you will let me, I would like to take you through a process that will allow you to be someone completely different in the future. Based on my failure to help anyone as the Food Nazi, I created an easy, loving way to help that works. Now they call me the "Food Prophet."

THE UN-DIET DEFINED: TIMELY,
EASY, AND AFFORDABLE

Amount (Food Volume)

Like most people, I need a diet in which I can eat all I want and still look and feel the way I want.

If you follow the Un-Diet perfectly, you can eat all you want. You only need to reduce quantities based on how far you deviate from the program.

Taste and Price

Typically, when you think of the things you are supposed to be shoveling into your mouth, you think, *Yucky—and pricey!* I was exactly the same way. That is why, for even the most inexperienced of healthy eaters, the food and meals I recommend in the Un-Diet taste good and are affordable. Like me, one day you will enjoy your Un-Diet more than your old diet and will spend less money following it.

Buying foods like fruits, fresh and frozen vegetables, jasmine rice, and potatoes in bulk is extremely cheap. Compared to eating out or purchasing prepackaged foods, even protein foods like eggs, chicken, salmon, canned tuna, and turkey are comparably affordable.

You'll find staple items such as flaxseed, almond milk, and almond butter in the health food store or health food section of the grocery store. Some of these items can get pricey, but they taste great, they are great for you, and they are worth it.

Health food stores also carry organic foods. Organic items, particularly meats, will help keep your diet more free of chemicals. However, organic food can be expensive and difficult to find.

Ease

My wife can shop for the week for my two children and me in about twelve minutes, with the occasional run to the health food store to reload. We enjoy eating at home so much more than going out now, based on taste and how good we look and feel eating this way.

We always cook several meals at a time. Chicken breasts, whole grain rice, sweet potatoes, and vegetables can be cooked in volume and used for several days.

When you go to work or travel, you can pack food in containers or bags to prevent hunger or being stuck in a place where there is nothing else to eat.

The Un-Diet Food Guide found on pages 82–84 easily explains when to eat carbohydrates, proteins, and fats—at the time God designed you to eat them.

FOOD BY GOD

When God developed the body, He specifically created certain foods for its use. These are the foods that grow and exist in nature. They are "Food by God." God has built into His foods everything that is necessary, in just the right amounts and in the perfect balance needed, for proper digestion, distribution, and elimination of nutrients.

The BBG digestive system is an intricate network of food-processing organs whose purpose is to break down and utilize the food you eat. Each component of the digestive system is so divinely complex that no human could ever truly create or even describe it. Every single part is a universe unto itself. All the organs of this system have unique cells, glands, fluids, and functions that are divinely formulated to play a specific role in the amazing manner in which the very demanding BBG processes food. When you take in Food by God in its natural state, the digestive system will easily break it down, dispense the nutrients to body cells, and quickly eliminate leftover toxins and by-products.

Food by God is packed with living vitamins, minerals, water, fiber, and the enzymes needed to digest the food itself. These, along with dozens of other elements we know about—and countless numbers of elements only God knows about—are what make up Food by God.

Owner's Manual Tip: Food by God Is "Smart Food"

Food by God and all the vitamins, minerals, and other elements it contains are put together by the intelligence of God. Food by God is smart food. When you eat Food by God, such as an apple or a carrot, it knows what to do inside the BBG, and the intelligent BBG knows what to do with it.

FOOD BY GOD LIST

The following is a selection of the most beneficial Foods by God:

Fruits

- Apples
- Bananas (High blood sugar effect)
- Blackberries
- Blueberries
- Cantaloupe
- Currants
- Grapefruit
- Grapes
- Honeydew melons
- Kiwi
- Lemons
- Limes
- Mangoes
- Nectarines
- Oranges
- Peaches
- Pears
- Pineapple
- Plums
- Prunes
- Raisins
- Raspberries
- Strawberries
- Tangerines
- Watermelon

Good Carbohydrates

- All-natural, whole-grain, chemical-free, sugar-free breads, flours, and cereals
- Barley
- Brown, jasmine, and basmati rice
- Buckwheat
- Cream of brown rice
- Grits
- Millet
- Oats
- Other hot whole-grain cereals (barley, quinoa, rye, spelt, millet, flax)
- Quinoa
- Rice cakes, rice noodles, puffed rice cereal
- Rye
- Spelt
- Unprocessed soy

Starchy Vegetables

- Corn
- Peas
- Potatoes
- Squash
- Sweet potatoes

Vegetables

- Alfalfa
- Artichokes
- Arugula
- Asparagus
- Bamboo shoots
- Beets
- Broccoli
- Brussels sprouts
- Cabbage
- Carrots
- Cauliflower
- Celery
- Collard greens
- Cucumbers
- Eggplant
- Escarole
- Green beans
- Kale
- Lettuce: All kinds
- Mesclun
- Mustard greens
- Onions
- Parsley
- Parsnips
- Pea pods
- Portabello
  mushrooms
- Radishes
- Radiccio
- Scallions
- Seaweed
- Shallots
- Swiss chard
- Snap peas
- Snow peas
- Spinach
- String beans
- Tomatos (also
  considered fruit)
- Turnips
- Watercress
- Wheat grass
- Zucchini

Beans (Protein and carbohydrate)

- Chickpeas
- Fresh Soy
- Kidney
- Lentil
- Lima
- Navy
- Pinto
- White

Nuts (Fat and protein)

- Almonds
- Brazil nuts
- Hazelnuts
- Pine nuts
- Walnuts

(These are all good for creating a healthy, more basic environment)

Seeds (Fat and protein)

- Flax
- Pumpkin
- Sesame
- Sunflower

Good Proteins

Eggs

- Best are from organic, free-range chickens

Fish

- Grouper
- Halibut
- Mackerel
- Mahimahi
- Rainbow trout
- Salmon
- Sardines
- Sea bass
- Snapper
- Swordfish
- Trout
- Tuna
- Whitefish

Poultry

- Chicken/turkey breast (Best from organic free-range)

Red Meat

- From organic, grass-fed beef
- Lean beef

Good Fats

- Almonds/Almond butter
- Avocados
- Crushed flaxseed (cold-pressed flaxseed oil can be used although not real stable)
- Extra-virgin coconut oil
- Fish oil
- Olives (Oil: cold-pressed, extra-virgin)
- Organic fats in grass- and vegetable-fed beef, egg yolks, and chicken
- Tahini (sesame and olive oil)
- Walnuts

Beverages

- Almond, rice, or oat milk
- Fresh fruit and vegetable juices
- Herbal tea
- Water: Reverse osmosis, distilled, fresh spring, filtered

Condiments

(Condiments are not used in heavy amounts so can do little damage, unless they are from a chemical source.)

- All-natural hot sauce
- Basil, curry, dill, garlic, ginger, horseradish, mint, miso, mustard, paprika, parsley, rosemary, tarragon, and thyme
- Butter Buds without hydrogenated oil
- Ginger
- High-quality vinegar
- Lemon juice
- Natural mustards
- Natural soy sauce or tamari
- Olive oil–based and low-fat, chemical-free dressings
- Sesame seeds
- Spices without MSG or hydrolyzed vegetable protein

Sweeteners

- Almond butter
- Brown rice syrup
- Fruit and fruit juice
- Honey
- Unrefined maple syrup
- Unsweetened, all-natural fruit jellies and syrups

FOOD BY MAN

"Food by Man" is food that is created or altered by man. It is also food that God did not design for the express purpose of being consumed or processed by your BBG on a regular basis.

The farther away you get from eating the foods God specifically created for the BBG, or the farther these foods are from their natural forms, the less efficiently the digestive system can break them down. If at all.

Food by Man is almost all indigestible. Because these foods cannot pass through the digestive system quickly and cannot be broken down well, they will linger inside your body. This will block the processing of other nutrients, rob you of power, contaminate your organs, create excess fat storage, affect your mood, and contribute to every type of symptom and disease known to humankind.

Food by Man lacks life or any truly usable vitamins, minerals, or other nutrients. Anything that is devoid of nutrition or life is unlikely to be able to *sustain* life.

There are many eating decisions you can make that are far from the best for your BBG's health and longevity. Fortunately, when working well, the digestive system is so incredible that it can break down and somehow utilize bad fuel sources. In addition, the body has multiple protective mechanisms for cleaning out toxins and restoring harmony, which can keep you alive or at least functioning.

Unfortunately, Food by Man will not allow you to function well or long.

Owner's Manual Tip: Food by Man Is Dumb

Food by Man is created by man and so does not contain any of God's intelligence. Therefore, it does not know what to do in the BBG, and the BBG has no idea what to do with it. Food by Man is "dumb." It is not smart to eat anything God did not make.

The Body by God #1 Nutrition Rule

The farther away any product is from its natural state, the way God made it, the more potentially harmful it is to the BBG. Therefore, these foods are highly likely to poison and damage your BBG and should definitely be considered "harmful if swallowed."

For example: aspartame, fast-food burgers and fries, sugar, dairy products like milk, cheese, and ice cream, and refined flour products like breads, pastries, and cereal are all foods far removed from their natural states.

ALL I EVER NEEDED TO KNOW ABOUT NUTRITION, I LEARNED IN JUNIOR HIGH

After traveling all over the world with the U.S. Olympic Team, I discovered very quickly that outside the United States, very few people are overweight. On my first trip to Europe, the only person I saw with a large belly was a gentleman in the airport wearing an "I LOVE NEW YORK" T-shirt!

The reality is, Americans do not actually eat *more* than the rest of the world. In fact, in much of Europe, food is an even larger part of their culture, and their diet contains even more rich and fattening foods. The problem is not that Americans eat more food. The problem is that we eat more Food by Man.

The excessive obesity and the extremely high rate of nutritionally related disease in Western society is related less to how much food Americans eat than to what is done to those foods. Health problems caused by food in the United States are mostly due to the fact that a high percentage of the American diet is made up of highly refined convenient and fast foods. These foods are prepared with an abundance of chemicals, additives, and preservatives, many of which are not even allowed in other parts of the world.

Outside America, meals are more often prepared fresh, from scratch and with actual foods, not synthetic convenience foods from a box or a package retrieved through a drive-up window.

Convenient, refined foods contain sugar-based and other types of chemical additives that make food impossible for your BBG to process or utilize. When food materials linger in the system, they cause damage to the organs, poison the body, block absorption of other nutrients, and get stored as a lot of excess baggage—fat.

$$A + B = C$$

Back in eighth-grade chemistry class, I learned the basic equation that is the foundation for the entire chemical world: $A + B = C$.

What this formula means is that when you take substance A and add it to substance B, it will equal substance C. It also means that if you take substance A, add it to substance B, and then add something else, such as P or S, you no longer get substance C. Instead, you get something entirely different: $A + B + S$ or $P = CS$ or CP.

For example, if you take 2 hydrogens and add 1 oxygen, you get H_2O, or water ($2H + 1O = H_2O$). However, if you take 2 hydrogens and add 2 oxygens, you no longer get water; you get hydrogen peroxide ($2H + 2O = H_2O_2$). You don't have to be a licensed nutritionist to realize that a glass of hydrogen peroxide is not nearly as nutritious—or refreshing—as a glass of water.

God has formulated your bloodstream in much the same way. A and B are all the essential, important, natural elements God has added to your body to create C. C is pure, life-giving blood; $A + B = C$ (pure, healthy blood). However, when you take in medications or chemicals and toxins found in the convenient, refined Food by Man, you now have A + B + XYZ = CXYZ or W or R or something other than the blood God designed you to have coursing through your BBG.

While in emergency situations some medications may be necessary, and it would be impossible to eliminate all chemicals, toxins, and Food by Man, their intake should be limited. Thankfully, the BBG is able to cleanse itself as long as the level of poisons is not too overwhelming.

Nutrition Formula for Health

When you take in un-man-ipulated, chemical-free Food by God, or FBG, the body more easily converts it into A and B. As a result, you are most likely to get clean, healthy C.

FBG + FBG = HEALTHY BBG

Warning: "Food by Man" may be hazardous to your health.

Owner's Manual Tip

If you fuel your body with Food by Man, the energy required to operate the digestive system becomes so great that power will be robbed from the other systems in the body. This is particularly dangerous because it will eventually weaken the BBG immune system.

Fueling with Food by God will minimize the amount of power needed for digestion, leaving *more power* for the rest of the body.

COMMON FOODS BY MAN

In 1 Corinthians 3:16–17, we are told that a body is one place where God lives: "Don't you know that you yourselves are God's temple and that God's Spirit lives in you? If anyone destroys God's temple, God will destroy him; for God's temple is sacred, and you are that temple." The Bible is saying that your Body by God is God's temple, and you should not poison, defile, or destroy it.

Your temple, your Body by God, was created to be kept as sacred and pure as possible. Food by Man is food that is toxic, full of chemicals, or does not belong in the system. That is why in the Old Testament many types of these foods are called "unclean."

Eating Food by Man on a regular basis is like going to your place of worship every day and tossing garbage and chemicals all over the altar of God's house. That's not right.

Following is a list of primary examples of man-made fuels, or Food by Man. These foods are far away from what God created and designed for the human body to consume and process:

FOOD BY MAN

The following is a selection of primary Foods by Man, which are *not* beneficial to your health:

- Pork
- Shellfish
- Sugar Substitutes
- Hydrogenated Oils
- Additives, Colorings, Flavorings, and Preservatives
- Fast, Refined, and Fried Foods
- Other Animal Products
- Dairy
- Caffeine
- Refined Sugar
- Table Salt
- White Foods

DO NOT CLOSE THE BOOK AFTER READING THIS LIST!

You do not have to avoid everything on this list to get healthier and look and feel better! While the Un-Diet teaches reducing these foods, it is more about adding better ones. I believe you will find that the Food by God I recommend is not only healthy, but can be enjoyable as well. While it may be challenging to reduce Food by Man in your diet, by following the Un-Diet Food Guide on pages 82–84 you will see remarkable improvements even while still eating the modern Food by Man diet.

Pork

Foods receiving poor ratings from God in the Bible are usually good ones to avoid putting in your mouth. In His infinite wisdom concerning all of life, health, and longevity, God mentions that "the pig . . . is unclean for you" (Lev. 11:7). Other animals referred to on this list are camels, dogs, and horses—all good animals to steer clear of consuming.

While eating meat from the wrong animals doesn't keep you out of heaven or make you a bad person, avoiding pork turns out to be a solid recommendation. Because pig tissues are so high in fat, their flesh absorbs many of the toxins and poisons they are exposed to as a result of their lifestyle.

Like all animal products, pork is high in saturated fat and cholesterol. The numerous pork by-products, such as ham, sausage, and bacon, are also heavily treated with salt, sugar, and various chemicals. This makes them additionally harmful to the digestive organs of your BBG fuel processing system.

As you ingest the meat and meat by-products of pigs, the poisons in their flesh, along with the dangers of consuming animal products and chemically treated foods, are unnaturally passed on to you.

Shellfish

The Bible also states, "Anything living in the water that does not have fins and scales is to be detestable to you" (Lev. 11:12). This is also sound wisdom, as shellfish are another of the foods most toxic to the Body by God's internal environment.

(Other animals on this list categorized alongside shellfish are eagles, vultures, ravens, owls, and insects.)

Fish droppings are the main diet of shellfish. Today, fish are exposed to the high

---

Old Testament Nutritional Advice for Today

I am sure that if eating the common Foods by Man existed at the time the Old Testament was being written, they would have been listed in the book of Leviticus as additional "unclean" foods to be avoided in order to keep your temple (body) holy.

level of chemicals now present in the earth's waters. The fish then excrete these chemicals in a concentrated form. These poisonous fish droppings are then consumed by shellfish such as crab, clams, mussels, and lobster, which are little more than the scavengers of the seafloor.

Like pork products, shellfish will literally pollute your body's ecosystem, defile your temple, and become hazardous to your health.

Sugar Substitutes

The taste for sugar is a craving shared by all. The problem is that sugar can be potentially harmful to your organs, lower your energy, affect your mood, rot your teeth, and cause you to gain fat when it is present in your food on a regular basis. The desire for this element is so great, however, that man has searched both land and laboratory for substitutes that imitate the pleasurable flavor of sugar but don't have the negative consequences.

This quest has resulted in several chemical experiments, creating formulas such as saccharine, aspartame, sucralose, sorbitol, maltodextrin, dextrose, and several other scary-sounding synthetic alternatives.

The digestive organs of your BBG fuel digesting system are highly sensitive. The effects that artificial materials will have on their function is extremely perilous. (Remember: A + B = C) You should now sense danger when it comes to ingesting any chemical alternatives such as these. In fact, these artificial materials are so dangerous that if a sugar substitute is added to a product, manufacturers must put a warning label on the package to alert health-conscious consumers.

Natural sweeteners (like honey or maple syrup) still in their natural states are the only ones designed by God to be consumed and assimilated by the living cells of the BBG. Only God's supernatural intelligence is capable of developing something that allows for completely safe consumption.

Any synthetic sweeteners created by a human being in a laboratory, or a natural sweetener that has been refined, modified, or changed, cannot properly move through the essential organs of digestion or react without error with the bloodstream. As a result, somewhere along the line, you will run into a health problem due to eating these products.

All sugar, salt, or fat substitutes of any kind are chemically based, highly refined, and created in a laboratory by men and not in nature by God. The first widely used sugar substitute was saccharine, also known as Sweet 'N Low. Large doses of this chemical concoction were found to cause cancer in laboratory animals. Anything promoting death in large doses cannot promote life or be healthy in small doses.

This discovery should have served as a warning of the toxic, pathological nature of chemical sweeteners. However, when the dangers of saccharine became known, rather than aborting further efforts to manipulate the human sweet tooth, scientists began looking for a saccharine substitute. Eventually, they created aspartame.

The diet product known as aspartame, or the name brand NutraSweet, is the one typically found in nearly all "sugar-free" products. Aspartame was chemically isolated in a laboratory, making aspartame no longer in its natural state and therefore no longer from God. This should issue an immediate warning to you that the effects of consuming aspartame can be unpredictable and potentially hazardous to your BBG.

Aspartame has an effect similar to that of two other Foods by Man: monosodium glutamate, otherwise known as MSG, and hydrolyzed vegetable proteins. None of these react well chemically within the organ systems and can actually be considered "chemical poisons." These compounds are extremely toxic to the brain and can cause serious chronic neurological disorders as well as a host of other symptoms.

Remember the Body by God #1 Nutrition Rule: *The farther away any product is from its natural state, the way God made it, the more potentially harmful it is to the BBG.* Artificial additives or chemically altered substances are actually the farthest away from any tree, river, field, or farm. Therefore, they are highly likely to poison and damage your BBG. Chemical sweeteners and seasonings should definitely be considered "harmful if swallowed."

Hydrogenated Oils

Hydrogenated and partially hydrogenated oils, which contain "trans-fatty acids," are created by an artificial processing of vegetable oils. This is done to retard spoilage and keep baked sweets and margarine from falling apart or melting at room temperature. Once again, any edible material that has been changed, altered, or distorted in any way is no longer intended for BBG use and is therefore unsafe. Because hydrogenated oils cannot be processed normally by the body, they negatively affects cholesterol levels and a certain percentage of all heart and circulatory disease every year is actually directly attributed to the intake of trans-fats.

Found in margarine, baked goods, and refined, fast, and packaged foods, hydrogenated oils are a common ingredient of the kind of quick snacks found in vending machines, fast-food restaurants, and convenience stores everywhere. If at all possible, they should be totally avoided.

Additives, Colorings, Flavorings, and Preservatives

The additives, colorings, flavorings, and preservatives introduced to modern food products and beverages are nothing more than pure chemical compounds. The effects of these chemicals over time cause serious damage to the BBG's delicate digestive system.

For the most part, the Body by God is unable to break down foods and drinks that have been refined with these toxic chemicals. As mentioned earlier, when food materials linger in the system, they cause damage to the organs, poison the body, block the absorption of nutrients, and make you fat.

Many colorings, additives, flavorings, and preservatives like sulfites, nitrites, nitrates, salicylates, propylene, and glycol are made up of the same materials as some of the chemicals you will find in household cleaners, in your medicine cabinets, or in maintenance products in your garage!

The disease, obesity, emotional problems, and learning disorders related specifically to the use of these compounds is prevalent mostly in the United States. That is because most such food additives are not even approved in other countries.

The risk factors here should be obvious. These are not only chemicals, but chemicals designed with the specific purpose of manipulating, preserving, and altering the matter of the products that contain them. They will have the same effect on the cells of your brain and body, and so should be approached with extreme caution.

Fast, Refined, and Fried Foods

Fast, refined, and fried foods such as hamburgers, fries, sodas, cookies, donuts, chips, fried chicken, and other greasy, refined, and especially packaged foods are extremely difficult, if not impossible, to process or digest. These highly fabricated, counterfeit foods are lacking any usable nutrition, are outrageously high in unhealthy types of fats, and contain many of the dangerous additives, colorings, flavorings, and preservatives mentioned earlier.

This is another case of foods that will linger in the system and cause harm. As a result, not only do they not supply you with any nourishment, they block your colon. This stops you from being able to absorb the foods that *do* have nutritional value.

These foods rob your delicate BBG systems of power. As a result, you become tired and fatigued, which is not a normal way to feel. Although it may *seem* "normal" if this is your typical diet and way of feeling.

The power being drained by these fast, refined, and impossible-to-process foods is taken directly from your BBG immune system and other organ functions. This will eventually lead to serious health complications and slow down or even stop the healing process. Refined, convenient foods are a leading contributor to all intestinal diseases, up to and including colon cancer.

In addition to the fat storage that results from all foods that stay in the digestive system, the fat, calorie, and carbohydrate levels of these foods are so incredibly high, excess fat is guaranteed to be deposited somewhere on your body. This type of "junk" food not only is harmful to the health of your BBG, but it is also the chief cause of your body's becoming enlarged.

OVERUSE OF ANIMAL PRODUCTS

Many lean animal products are part of the guidelines for fueling found in your *Owner's Manual* Un-Diet program. However, for the following reasons, they should be eaten only as recommended.

Fruits and vegetables are the true Food by God. You can pull them right off the tree or right out of the ground and eat them "as is." Their fleshy tissues are alive and packed with high-quality vitamins, minerals, enzymes, and other nutrients, all packed in water. Because your BBG is also living and made up of mostly water, the human body effortlessly absorbs these nutrients when eaten according to the Un-Diet Food Guide. The "living waters" present in these foods are God's perfect meal.

The high fiber content of fruits and vegetables allows for unused elements to swiftly exit the body. On the opposite end of the food processing spectrum are animals. Animal flesh is dry, fiber-less, and like all Food by Man—dead.

In truth, God did not design your BBG to be a carnivore, or meat eater. Completely different from humans, carnivores such as dogs, lions, and grizzly bears have large fangs, claws, and a digestive system designed specifically for the task of absorbing meat. They are also able to eat their meat raw, when it is not dried out and the enzymes needed for processing it are still living. However, you should not eat raw meat. Your BBG digestive system is not equipped to appropriately break down this uncooked meat or to deal with the high levels of germs and bacteria that are present within the flesh.

The fact that you must cook meat thoroughly to avoid contracting a disease from some deadly organism living inside should also indicate to you that the overuse of animal products can be harmful.

In addition to the animal flesh itself, the very source of animal products creates an additional pitfall. The chickens, pigs, turkeys, and cows we get our meat and milk from are typically not out roaming free in nature as God intended. Instead, today's commercial animal product farms are more like factories.

To speed up production and avoid dealing with health issues, commercial animals are fed and injected with large amounts of antibiotics, steroids, drugs, and hormones. Unless you raise or hunt your own animals, the meat is neither clean nor created by God. Instead, it is manufactured, and tainted, by man. For this reason, if you can, attempt to get organically raised grass and vegetable-fed meats and animal products.

While animals raised naturally, eating grass and vegetables, contain healthier types of fats, meat from commercially grown animals contains saturated fat and is high in cholesterol. When saturated fats and cholesterol are present in high levels in the bloodstream, they will settle in and begin to block the arteries and vessels that carry blood to and from the heart. This is yet another reason to eat only the foods recommended in your Owner's Manual.

The rough, fatty flesh of meat, particularly red meat, along with the high saturated fat content, makes it extremely hard to break down and fully process. Putting large amounts of meat into your system will create all the hazards and disease associated with foods that do not pass through the digestive organs quickly and easily.

As a result, inappropriate or overuse of animal products should be avoided to extend the life of your BBG.

Dairy Products

In addition to the perils of the other animal products already discussed, dairy products are in a whole new category of man-made foods. God designed dairy products for a completely different animal. Cow's milk was created for cows. In fact, realistically, it was not even created for cows, but for *baby* cows.

While milk was created by God (for calves), I've always wondered who was the first person to bend over, look under the cow, and say, "I'm going to start sucking on those things and if it tastes good, I'm going to put it in my coffee."

In addition to being intended for an entirely different species, cow's milk has to go through a processing and refining system known as "pasteurization" in order to make it safe to use for drinking and cooking. The fact that milk must be treated before human consumption should already be an indicator to you that it is not something you should regularly ingest.

During this treatment, the milk is heated to kill off germs. Unfortunately, when something is heated in this manner, not only are the germs destroyed, but so are many of the nutrients, as well as the enzymes necessary for digesting the nutrients.

A calf cannot survive on this refined milk. Neither can a human. In fact, dairy products are a leading cause of allergic reactions and create a tremendous amount of malfunction in the BBG.

The milk from a cow is designed for the specific purpose of adding several hundred pounds to the size of its offspring in a short period of time. In order to accomplish this enormous task, "calves' milk" is made up of a high percentage of proteins, and the size of these proteins is extremely large. Contrary to that, human breast milk was created with the goal of adding only a couple of dozen pounds to children in a similar period of time. Therefore, "human milk" has a much lower concentration of protein, and the size of the proteins are much smaller by comparison.

As you get older, your BBG is less equipped to break down milk. It appears that God did not design adult humans, or any other mature animal for that matter, to consume milk. This makes sense, because as you grow it gets harder to stick your head under a cow.

Contrary to popular belief, milk and dairy products do not give you strong bones. Due to pasteurization and the fact that the nutrients in cow's milk were meant for calves, the calcium in milk and dairy products cannot be efficiently used by humans for bone growth. Additionally, dairy products create a dangerous acidic environment* in

---

*See "Back to Basics" on page 76.

the body. The results of this acidic condition cause deterioration of the delicate bone tissue. This makes dairy products *bad* for bone growth, instead of good for it.

Potentially, the most dangerous part of dairy consumption, however, is the treatment of the cows themselves. As mentioned previously, cows are fed and injected with a host of antibiotics, drugs, steroids, and hormones during their lives. A portion of these chemicals and poisons will naturally end up in the milk these cows produce, and eventually on top of your cereal.

If you choose to use dairy products, buy raw, organic items from a farm, health food store, or special service if possible.

Fortunately for you and your Body by God, it is quite possible to obtain a significant amount of calcium *without* dairy products, by eating plenty of green leafy vegetables (Where do you think cows get it from?) and other calcium-rich foods actually created for *your* species.

Rice and almond milk make excellent replacements for cow's milk. They are natural, taste sweeter than milk, and can be found in health food stores and most grocery stores.

Caffeine

Caffeine is a common stimulant found in everything from chocolate, coffee, and soda to vitamins, herbs, and medication. Many people use it to raise their normal energy levels in the morning. This process is repeated to keep them awake throughout the day, so that by the next morning it has to be started all over again.

The problem is that God designed your BBG to stay balanced. The body is always seeking what is called *homeostasis,* or a natural, God-given balance of function and physiology. If you drink or swallow something that elevates the body's power level, you cause a disturbance in this balance, and the body tries to save itself by bringing power levels back down. Over time, your Body by God keeps adjusting its natural power state downward to compensate for this overstimulation.

That is why it eventually takes more and more caffeine to give you any effect. Sooner or later you have to drink a cup of coffee just to get back to "tired."

Like all stimulants, every time you drink caffeine, you affect your heart function, alter your vascular flow, and overstimulate digestive and glandular activity. Anytime you manipulate your BBG in any way, you end up throwing off your normal energy balance, which will eventually cause organ system failure and glandular meltdown.

The regular use of caffeine or any material that speeds up body function will ultimately slow it down.

Refined Sugar

Sugar comes from the sugarcane plant, which grows in nature. But in order to create the sugar you find in all packaged foods, food additives, white packets, and on your kitchen table, these natural plants go through intensive refining. The refining process turns sugar into a concentrated chemical without any nutritional worth that is far removed from its natural state as a plant.

As with any chemical, when sugar is ingested by your body it can create negative overreactions by the glands and many of the organs, as well as altering the very physiology of the brain. Depression, thought dysfunction, diabetes, and dozens of other disorders all can be linked to the use of sugar on a regular basis. Because excess sugar is stored as fat, refined sugar is also a leading cause of obesity.

When you ingest a chemical like sugar, it can have the same effect as any addictive drug. Your BBG defense system's organs of immunity react to sugar in the same manner as they react to tobacco, marijuana, cocaine, alcohol, and many other drugs or allergens—by forming antibodies against it. Simply put, these antibodies will then continuously crave the chemical and, as a result, you form a physical addiction to sugar.

When it comes to sugar, it is best to try to break the habit.

Table Salt

Table salt is another refined food, and so by definition is also no longer fit for human consumption. The highly acidic nature of refined salt and the high concentration of sodium it contains negatively affect the body's physiology and stress the cardiovascular system, the digestive system, the kidneys, the skeletal system, and other organs of the BBG.

"White" Foods

The "white" foods are white rice and foods made from white flour, such as white bread, pastries, and white pasta. White foods have all been so massively refined by modern food production that there is no nutrition left to be absorbed by your Body by God. All the fiber, vitamins, minerals, and other nutrients needed for good health have been taken out. Therefore, white foods offer no benefit to your internal cells and systems.

Much like fried foods or other heavily refined consumables, white foods move slowly through the digestive system and block the intestines. Once again, this stops you from absorbing and eliminating nutrients and delays proper processing. This leaves the BBG vulnerable to intestinal illnesses, weight gain, fatigue, allergies, toxicity, and colon cancer associated with foods that hinder the function of your digestive organs.

The next time someone asks you to put a white food in your mouth, say that you might as well put it in the other end—because that is where it will end up getting *stuck* anyway.

5 | UNDERSTANDING THE DIFFERENT TYPES OF FUELS

Food can be broken down into three major categories: carbohydrates, proteins, and fats. Within these categories are the nutrients God created as raw materials to make up the BBG, and which are necessary for it to survive. Nutrients include vitamins, minerals, amino acids, enzymes, and many other accessory elements we know about— and countless elements only God knows about.

Each category affects the body in a different way. By understanding these effects, you will comprehend what foods God created for you to eat and when you should eat them.

CARBOHYDRATES

Carbohydrates were designed to be broken down into sugar and used for power by the body. Unrefined Food by God containing carbohydrates slowly converts to sugar in the system for safe, sustained levels of power.

Carbohydrate power is used as "fire" in the normal fat-burning process inside the body. An important effect of taking in carbohydrates is that a certain amount of carbohydrates are responsible for holding water inside the body tissues.

Carbohydrates are also muscle sparing. Without carbohydrates, the body would eventually have to catabolize, or break down, its own muscles for energy.

A simple definition: Everything that does not have a mother, a face, or go to the bathroom is typically some part of the carbohydrate category.

See Chapter 4 for a list of Foods by God that contain good carbohydrates.

FRUITS AND VEGETABLES

When fruits and vegetables are eaten at the right time of day and in the right amounts—according to the Un-Diet Food Guide—they are the ideal Food by God. You can pull them right off the tree or pluck them right out of the ground and eat them "as is." (Of course, now you have to wash them—but they're still pretty close to perfect.)

The fleshy tissues of fruits and vegetables are made up of mostly water. This water is packed with high-quality living vitamins, minerals, antioxidants, enzymes, and other nutrients.

Because your BBG is also living and made up of mostly water, the human body effortlessly absorbs these valuable nutrients. Their high-fiber content then allows for the unwanted elements to swiftly exit the body. The "living waters" present in these foods are God's perfect meal.

Apple vs. Broccoli	
Fruits	Vegetables
Increase blood sugar	Little blood sugar effect
Many carbohydrates	Few carbohydrates
Potentially yeast-forming	Non–yeast-forming and potentially yeast-fighting

Because fruit contains a significant amount of carbohydrates and sugar, it is best eaten only in the morning and does not combine well with other foods. Vegetables, on the other hand, are great to eat anytime or with almost anything.

Follow the BBG Un-Diet directions to make the best use of the two top Foods by God in the carbohydrate category.

Starchy Vegetables. Starchy vegetables like potatoes, sweet potatoes, squash, corn, and peas are almost as perfect as fruits and regular vegetables. They, too, are pulled or plucked. The only thing that makes them different is that they must be cooked, and they have a more considerable influence on blood sugar levels.

Note: Yams are loaded with good, colorful antioxidants and have a more moderate effect on blood sugar than regular potatoes, making them part of the Food by God all-star team.

Beans. Fresh beans are God-made foods that contain not only carbohydrates but also clean proteins. These are healthy foods when fresh and used according to the BBG Un-Diet guidelines.

WHOLE GRAINS

When eaten in their most natural state, whole grains such as brown, basmati, and jasmine rice, oats, rye, or barley are excellent BBG carbohydrate category food sources. All these foods are by God and contain many high-quality, readily usable nutrients.

Real whole grains, right off the farm, still contain the shell and all their original fiber and nutrients. They will take anywhere from twenty minutes to one hour to cook. The longer a grain takes to cook, the more whole it typically is.

The Whole Grain Rule: Farmed, Not Refined

The Whole Grain Rule states: "The less refined and the more whole (the closer to the farm) the grain is, the more properly it is processed inside the body and the more nutrients it still contains."

Whole-Grain Breads, Cereals, and Pasta. Whole grain breads, cereal, and pasta are the best man-made foods in the carbohydrate category because they are the closest to their natural state. However, they are at least partially refined and so are not broken down as properly and efficiently as unrefined whole grains.

These foods still contain some fiber and many usable nutrients but are highly concentrated carbohydrates. The less refined they are and the less that is added to them, the better.

Refined Grains, Cereals, Pastas (White Foods)

Remember the Whole Grain Rule. White foods are very refined and far from the farm. As a result, these types of carbohydrates lack nutrients and cannot be properly processed by the body. The more refined or chemically treated these products are, the more problems they can create inside the BBG.

Owner's Manual Tip: The Use of Grains in Your Feed Bag

Whole, close-to-the-farm grains are mostly healthy. However, they should be limited according to the Un-Diet plan due to the blood sugar and acid-causing* effects they have on the BBG.

Gluten found in wheat and wheat products is a common cause of food sensitivity reactions in the BBG that cause things like yeast infections, inflammatory bowel conditions, skin problems, and reflux. Therefore, they may need to be drastically reduced or eliminated in some Un-Diets.

*See Back to Basics on page 76.

Sugar (and Anything with Sugar in It)

While all other carbohydrates must be broken down into sugar by the body to enter the bloodstream, when straight sugars are consumed, they are dumped right in. This causes a meteoric rise in blood sugar, which stresses the entire BBG system.

With the sudden rise in blood sugar that straight sugar causes, the glands and certain other organs go into a state of alert and start doing everything they can to bring the blood sugar level back down. You get a quick spike up, then the sugar level comes plummeting back down, usually to below normal. Rather than giving you *more* power, the result of eating sugar ends up being *less* power.

There are different types of sugars, such as white, brown, and high-fructose corn syrup, cane, raw, honey, and fruit. White, brown, and high-fructose corn syrup are all refined and found in most artificial, convenient, and fast foods.

Cane, raw, and other less-refined sugars still provide an *unhealthy* high dose of concentrated sugar. Because they are closer to their God-given form, the body can react to them and process them somewhat better than sugar.

The natural sugar in fruit and honey is straight from God as long as it has not been refined or removed from the fruit. As a result, it is the most safely and easily utilized of all the sugars and contains some actual nutritional value.

Caution: Too Many Carbohydrates

While the carbohydrate family contains more natural, godly foods and is the best nutritional source for power, too many carbohydrate foods can cause health problems in the Body by God. An overabundance of carbohydrates loads the system with sugar, even if the carbohydrates come from a healthy source.

The high levels of blood sugar created by eating too many carbohydrates can cause pancreatic and glandular dysfunction, as well as blood and brain chemistry problems. This will stress the entire BBG and can lead to a host of symptoms, dysfunction, and disease.

An additional danger of an overabundance of carbohydrates in the BBG is that unused sugar power will be stored as fat, thus causing problems in the arteries, high blood pressure, high cholesterol, and other major health issues. So even though most carbohydrates are basically fat- and cholesterol-free, they *can* end up causing fat gain and a rise in cholesterol.

While we need foods in the carbohydrate category for power, few of us need *that much* power. Carbohydrate energy input should occur only in direct proportion to how much energy you put out. In fact, if you consume more energy food than you need, it actually ends up causing you to have *less* power.

With power foods, timing is everything. In the morning, or before or directly after strenuous exercise, there is a higher need for carbohydrate fuels. However, during periods of inactivity or just prior to sleeping, there is little need to consume carbohydrates, especially in mass quantities.

The tendency in many diets is to eat meals containing a lot of foods in the carbohydrate category just before bedtime. This creates an unhealthy situation by providing enough carbohydrates in the system to fuel running two NYC marathons, yet the person is going to bed and not using any power at all.

As a result, the system becomes challenged by all the issues resulting from an overabundance of unused carbohydrate sugar power in the system. Not only is this unhealthy, but the body has to work so hard all night just digesting it all that the individual wakes up feeling more tired than when he went to bed.

The Body by God Un-Diet along with the Un-Diet Food Guide will provide you with guidelines for safe, proper, and effective carbohydrate consumption.

PROTEINS

On the opposite end of the spectrum from carbohydrates is the protein category. Proteins are found in all foods, but are found most abundantly in animal products.

Animal protein is the most abundant source of amino acids, but it is not a good source of power. Most of the body's tissues are actually made up of protein. The amino acids present in protein foods are used for building, healing, and repairing these tissues.

Animal Protein

The most concentrated source of protein is animal flesh and animal products. Animal proteins contain the complete line of amino acids, as well as vitamin B_{12}, which is an essential nutrient for BBG function.

Also, animal proteins don't cause a rise in blood sugar, which is of significant benefit to BBG health and longevity.

Nuts, Seeds, Beans, Whole Grains, and Vegetables

Raw nuts and seeds, fresh beans, whole grains, and vegetables are less concentrated sources of protein. There is less protein and fewer amino acids present in these foods, but they are also healthy, natural, and a good source of carbohydrates and other important nutrients.

Combining these foods with other foods can give them the complete amino acid line they lack. Beans, peas, lentils, and unrefined soy combined with either whole grains or nuts and seeds will give you all the amino acids you need for healthy, Food by God concentrated protein. Soybeans contain a more complete protein, but are difficult to find unrefined in their natural state.

Caution: Too Much Protein

The lack of a clean source, the amount of drugs used on commercial animals, and the chemicals used in refined proteins make high-protein diets toxic and hard on the immune system.

Overuse of animal products falls into the Food by Man category, which is prone to creating all the problems associated with stepping away from the things God created for us to eat on a consistent basis.

Proteins and Carbohydrates Don't Digest Well Together

The process necessary to digest carbohydrates is different from the process used to digest protein. Proteins and carbohydrates also have contradicting effects on the internal environment of the BBG. As a result, ingesting large quantities of both carbohydrates and proteins at the same time will make it difficult for the body to break down and absorb either of them efficiently.

Meals should have either a carbohydrate focus, a protein focus, or a very moderate combination of both. Eating large portions of carbohydrates and proteins together, or eating them together too often, can create all the problems related to overworking or clogging up the digestive organs of the BBG fuel processing system.

Do Not Combine: Eggs and fruit, fruit and vegetables, meat and potatoes, spaghetti and meatballs, eggs and toast and hash browns, pepperoni and pizza, bread and meat, etc. All these combinations provide too many carbohydrates with too many proteins at once and cause disastrous collisions inside the fuel processing system.

FATS

Do you want the skinny on fats? Fats from animal, nut, seed, and vegetable sources are something that your brain needs for proper structure, your cells need for healthy function, and your glands need for balanced hormone production. Fats supply insulation and protection for the organs of the BBG, help store and transport fat-soluble vitamins (A, D, E, and K), assist in mineral absorption, and cause fat mobilization.

Fats will also reduce hunger signals to the feeding system, as you will tend to feel more full after eating them than you will after eating any of the other food categories. An additional benefit is that fats slow food absorption, which will allow for better blood sugar control, glandular activity, and weight loss.

Good Fats

Omega-3 Fatty Acids. Omega-3 fatty acids have been found to be the fats the BBG gets the best benefits from. These fats tend to produce the type of health fats are *supposed* to produce. They have been found to be beneficial for cardiovascular, joint, and immune system function.

Omega-3 fats are found in fish, fish oils, naturally raised grass- and vegetable-fed animals, flaxseed, and walnuts.

Good fish sources of omega-3 include salmon, sardines, mackerel, halibut, cod, and tuna. (Regrettably, eating fish must be limited due to the lack of a nontoxic food source, so fish oil will need to be taken by supplement.)

Other Good Fats. Although they are not omega-3 fats, the fats in almonds and Evening Primrose Oil have health-producing benefits. Almonds are basic pH producers, making them helpful for balancing the typical acidic diet. (See "Back to Basics" on page 76.) Evening primrose oil, along with the oil in flaxseed, supplies elements that help balance hormonal production.

Other good sources of fats are extra-virgin olive oil, coconut oil (a good saturated fat), and avocados. Cook using olive oil or coconut oil only. Olive oil is monounsaturated and coconut is saturated so they will not turn rancid or oxidize when heated. This allows for stability under heat, making them safe and healthy for use.

Fats to Reduce and Avoid

Other Omega Fats. Modern diets contain high levels of other omega fats. These other fats do not provide the same health-producing benefits as omega-3 fats, and because they are so abundant in our diets can have a harmful, inflammatory effect on many BBG systems. These damaging fats are found in processed foods, commercial meats, as well as vegetable, nut, and seed oils.

Saturated Fats. Saturated fats are the fats found in commercially raised animal products, palm, and coconut oil. While saturated fats contain certain benefits, an overabundance of these fats will harm the body and so should be limited. (Coconut oil contains several helpful properties and is a good, stable source of cooking oil.)

Vegetable, Nut, Bean, and Seed Oils. Vegetable, nut, bean, and seed oils are very unstable and break down into substances that are no longer healthy for the body, particularly when exposed to heat. The worst oils are the trans-fat- containing hydrogenated and partially hydrogenated oils as noted in the "Food by Man" section. These oils are vegetable oils that have been artificially altered so that they are unable to be used or easily broken down inside the body. These unprocessed fats end up being stored in dangerous and unwanted places.

Bad Fats

- Fats found in fried, greasy, fast foods
- Hydrogenated oils (Trans-Fats)
- Milk fat/cream
- Nongrass-, nonorganic-fed animal fats
- Palm oils
- Vegetable oils removed from original source

Caution: Too Much Fat

Be careful with fat. Too much fat, even *good* fat, will make you fat. Fat has the largest amount of calories of all the food categories. Therefore, eating too many fats or consuming Food by Man that contains added fat is most likely to be left unused and put aside as fat.

COMBINING FATS WITH CARBOHYDRATES AND PROTEINS: *THE GOOD, THE BAD, AND THE UGLY*

Adding fats to your meals is essential. Nonetheless, due to their high concentration of calories and the importance of not accumulating fat in your body, combining fats with carbohydrates, proteins, or both should be approached with extreme caution.

When you eat carbohydrates alone, without fats or protein, large or concentrated amounts of sugar will be dumped into your system. This will cause the pancreas to secrete large amounts of insulin in order to contain and bring down blood sugar levels, which will create strain on several organs of the body, fatigue, and lead to higher levels of body fat. You will also crave carbohydrates and sugar as a response to the low blood sugar effects created by the insulin.

By adding small amounts of fats and or small amounts of proteins to carbohydrate meals, you can help to create more gradual carbohydrate digestion.

The Good

Small amounts of proteins and/or fats with a larger serving of carbohydrates.

A small amount of a healthy fat, a small serving of protein, or a very small serving of both eaten with a carbohydrate will help slow down the rise in blood sugar and stop the oversecretion of insulin by the pancreas. *This is especially helpful if your BBG has blood sugar issues.*

For example: 1 egg (protein) with oatmeal (carbohydrate) sweetened with a teaspoon of almond butter (good fat), toast with extra-virgin olive oil drizzled on it, and ground flaxseed sprinkled on a sweet potato. (If you have ever had olive oil on your bread in an Italian restaurant, you know that olive oil and flaxseed oil taste really good on carbohydrates. You also know one of the many reasons Europeans have less heart disease than Americans.)

Or: Larger serving of proteins with moderate amount of fats.

For example: salmon (protein/good fat) Caesar salad with avocados (good fat) and olives (good fat), or chicken, cashews, and broccoli stir-fried in extra-virgin olive oil, and a 1-egg-yolk/4-egg-white omelette cooked in a skillet that is greased with coconut oil.

The Bad

Large amounts of fat with larger servings of carbohydrates.

Simply put, this will make you fat.

For example: pizza, linguini Alfredo, donuts, pancakes, hash browns, cookies, bread and butter, and a loaded potato.

And the Ugly

Too much of all three.

Too many fats, carbohydrates, and proteins together should always be eaten in the presence of a physician trained in CPR or close to a hospital. These are called "heart-explosion meals." After eating like this, you will most likely see a significant rise in pulse rate, blood pressure, and cholesterol by the end of the meal.

For example: steak-and-cheese sub, eggs and pancakes with butter and syrup, or a cheeseburger and French fries.

Body by God Owner's Fat Tip: Get Skinny on Fat

The concept of eating fat-free is not only unhealthy, it may also cause you to get fat. Good fats like those found in flaxseed, olives, and fish help the body mobilize stored fats. Additionally, the body must take in fat to stay adept at absorbing and utilizing it. Adding small to moderate amounts of good fats to healthy, low-fat Food by God will help the BBG to function better and actually make it leaner.

BACK TO BASICS:

Basics Are Good to the Bone but Acids Are Bad to the Bone

The tissues and organs of the body tend to flourish in a more basic pH environment versus a more acidic pH environment. Being acidic is just as threatening as it sounds. You are literally burning, boiling, or melting your cells.

As your *Owner's Manual* has shown, the typical modern diet of flour, dairy products, sugar, and meat is dangerous for multiple reasons. One major reason is that this type of eating creates high levels of acid in the body.

Acidic blood can create most of the adverse health issues related to aging, especially bone loss and arthritic degeneration. The reason for this is that normally your kidneys attempt to keep the BBG basic by eliminating excess acids. However, regular consumption of acid-producing foods will result in an acid level too high for the kidneys to manage efficiently.

To reduce acid levels, the body needs to add bases. Bases neutralize or reduce the dangerous acid effect. When acid levels get too high, the body must attempt to neutralize these acids by dumping some bases into the blood stream. The best acid neutralizers in the body are calcium phosphate and calcium carbonate from bones. These bone elements are exemplary bases for counteracting dietary acids. As a result, bone is literally being washed away in a pool of acid.

Other effects of acidic blood include organ disruption and brain and artery damage and decay.

Commercial dairy products, flour, sugar, and caffeine are the most significant acid-producing culprits. Additionally, all animal products create acid in the system. These are all part of the Food by Man list, proving once again that nothing God did not specifically create to be eaten by your BBG will serve to make it better when eaten in large quantities.

Although they are high-quality Foods by God, whole grains and fruits are also somewhat acid-producing and so should be eaten only as recommended in the Body by God Un-Diet program.

On the other hand, vegetables are incredibly good at creating a more basic environment. By adding all the vegetables you can handle to your diet, you will help to stabilize the acids and allow your joints and other organs to heal or remain in good health.

Other good acid-neutralizing foods are fats like almonds, avocados, and flaxseed. Drinking a lot of clean water is also an essential part of creating a healthy, basic bodily environment.

WATER

All the food categories are important. But while the BBG can go weeks without food, it cannot go long without water before suffering some malfunction of all its operating systems. In fact, after only a few days without water, the entire BBG can shut down completely.

Your Body by God is made up of mostly water. If you took the water out of your body, you would basically be powder. The quality of the fluid that all your body's cells are made up of and resting in is largely determined by the quality of the fluids you are ingesting.

Sources of poor drinking water such as impure tap water, coffee, or soda dilute the quality of water in the body with chemicals, additives, and heavy metals.

Clean water is extremely necessary for continuously flushing out the toxins and acids you are consuming and producing every day. For clean sources of drinking water, remember this simple BBG Water Consumption Rule: You should never drink anything you wouldn't take a bath in.

The BBG Water Consumption Rule

You should never drink anything you wouldn't take a bath in.

To keep your internal hydration system running at peak efficiency—and to have enough fluid for your cells to thrive in—you need to drink plenty of water. Furthermore, your water should contain 2 Hs, an O, and as little else as possible!

While it is highly unlikely that you would ever drink too *much* water, it is very likely that you might not drink *enough*.

The BBG Water Drinking Health Tip

The combination of drinking plenty of water and focusing on a more basic diet will help in recovering or sparing the bones and joints of your BBG. Always remember: *A dry joint is an unhappy joint.*

CHOPPING AWAY AT JOINT PAIN

Poor health conditions are often due to poor food choices. When people start eating better foods, I have seen improvement, or even total recovery from, nearly every illness that exists.

Joint problems, in particular, are often associated with the regular use of acid-causing foods. One of the most intriguing characters I ever worked with was an Englishman in his late thirties who was a former world karate champion. He retired several years before seeing me due to severe arthritis in his knees and shoulders.

After learning about the acid-effects of certain staples in his diet like cheese, chocolate, coffee, tea, and red meat, he decided to consume them only on special occasions. Since none of the best doctors in Europe could help him, he really did not think simply changing his diet would help his arthritis. Nonetheless, since he had nothing to lose, he decided to try it.

The results of this study were nothing short of a miracle. Within just a few weeks of eliminating these foods, his joint pain had almost completely disappeared. The problems in his knees and shoulders would come back only when he put the acid foods back in his diet.

He immediately went back to training and competing in karate. Later that year he won the karate world championships again.

Using the Un-Diet along with a focus on a more basic diet, I have seen many patients see incredible results with arthritis, fibromyalgia, and other painful conditions of the joints and muscles.

NUTRIENTS BY GOD: "NUTRIENT COMMUNION"

Vitamins, minerals, amino acids, antioxidants, and all the other accessory nutrients we know about—and all the ones only God knows about—are the building blocks of the various parts of the BBG. These are all found in the major food categories and are needed for the health and longevity of all your organs and operating systems.

There are many nutrition programs that tout the wonders of vitamins, the miracles of minerals, and the healing powers of enzymes, tree bark, and fish noses. While the intake of certain nutrients is essential, and many of them can be catalysts to healing, for these important nutrients to be used most effectively, if at all, you must attempt to get them from foods in their most *natural* state.

In order to truly absorb a nutrient, the body needs a specific amount of all the other things God put inside the food the nutrient comes from. This is called synergy or "Nutrient Communion."

For example, vitamin A is an important nutrient the body needs to function properly. However, if you simply swallow vitamin A processed into a pill, you will not be able to use it properly or at all. This is because a man-made pill lacks Nutrient Communion. On the other hand, when consumed in a carrot, beta-carotene is converted to vitamin A inside the body and can be absorbed safely, efficiently, and effectively. This is because God placed a perfect balance of all the elements and nutrients inside a carrot that are necessary for the body to use vitamin A.

Similarly, the calcium in green leafy vegetables, sesame seeds, and unprocessed soy products was placed there by God with all the Nutrient Communion necessary to be completely and safely absorbed by humans—unlike cow's milk, in which God placed calcium with the Nutrient Communion needed for total absorption by a cow.

Refining and overcooking destroy Nutrient Communion. High-quality vitamins and minerals may be plentiful in fruits, vegetables, and fresh squeezed juices, but when you refine and pasteurize them into other products, or literally cook the juice out of them, they lose the ability for the body to effectively absorb the nutrients. In other words, flaxseed oil might be good for you, but it is best utilized when still in the flax.

Vitamins A, C, E, beta-carotene, and the mineral selenium have been found to be nutrients needed particularly by the immune and cardiovascular systems. These vitamins and minerals are important in the prevention of cancer and disease. An abundance of fruits and vegetables containing these important compounds—with Nutrient Communion—will provide for extended heart health and stronger immunity.

However, too much of any of these vitamins in an isolated supplement form—*without* Nutrient Communion—can actually be poisonous to the body or block the absorption of some of the other vitamins. As a result, taking vitamins could actually *cause* what you were trying to *prevent*.

Nutrient Communion cannot be created in a laboratory. Only Food by God that has not been changed by man contains the Nutrient Communion that is critical for the safe and reliable absorption and utilization of all nutrients.

> **IMPORTANT:** Nutrient *supplements* are critical due to the significant unlikelihood that anyone will eat enough of the right foods on a regular basis to obtain all the nutrients necessary for good health. But, supplements are just that, they are supplemental or in addition to taking in the right nutrients in the form of food. Supplements cannot replace the real nutrients found only in God-made food.

It has been shown that it is vital to take in high-quality vitamin, mineral, and omega-3 oil supplements daily. It is typically necessary to purchase quality supplements from a health-food store or a natural health-care provider's office. These locations can assist you in determining the correct amounts of nutrients to take and help you decide whether or not you need additional supplementation to deal with conditions that are a result of a lifetime of nutrient deficiency.

But remember, do not rely entirely on supplements as your only source of nutrients. Chasing health "nutrient by nutrient" is confusing, contradictory, and will most likely get you nowhere. Only Food by God can be the source of real nutrition, but supplements will definitely help.

FOODS AND VITAMINS DON'T HEAL

If you get to the scene of an accident and you find two victims, one who is dead and one who is just hanging on, who has a chance of making it? Obviously, only the one who is just hanging on. If you pour vitamins, minerals, herbs, apples, and drugs into the dead guy, he is still dead. Only the person who still has life in his body has a chance to recover. That is because foods, or anything else found outside the BBG, don't heal. Only the BBG can heal from within.

In fact, BBGs do not even heal. The deceased BBG may have as many or more organs inside than the live one, but it still can't heal. So, technically, BBGs don't heal either. What heals is not the BBG, but rather God's power *inside* of the BBG. Without His power, your BBG is nothing more than about $1.86 worth of dust and inert molecules.

So, vitamin C or any other letter of the alphabet is not a "cure" for the common cold. Yet the Body by God defense system's organs of immunity do require vitamin C and many other nutrients to keep you well—or get you well after you've been sick. Consequently, when you take vitamin C, the vitamin C doesn't heal you, it just provides the nourishment necessary so that God's power within your Body by God can heal you.

6 | THE WAY GOD DESIGNED YOU TO EAT: THE *UN*-DIET FOOD GUIDE

USING THE FOOD GUIDE

The Un-Diet Food Guide is the key to unlocking the age-old mystery of eating properly. It is the premier part of the Un-Diet program.

By focusing on the right food categories (carbohydrates, proteins, and fats) at the right times of day you will see miraculous things begin to occur both inside and outside your BBG. Remarkably, you will see this happen even if you do not eat ideal Food by God.

If you have any issues or conditions with your health, your weight, or your physical appearance, you will see drastic improvements simply by eating according to the Un-Diet Food Guide.

Eating Food by God is important. However, eating the way God designed you to eat can be of equal or even greater importance. For maximum BBG health and beauty, it is important not only to *eat more of what God wants you to eat,* but to *eat when He wants you to eat it.*

Following this Food Guide is so effective that even if you do not change the foods you eat but just eat them when you are supposed to according to the guide, you will see remarkable results in how you look and feel.

The Un-Diet Food Guide is based on the different needs for carbohydrates, protein, and fats the BBG has throughout the day. These needs are as follows:

Serving Size Key

HIGH = 2+ Servings
MODERATE = 1 to 2 Servings
LOW = .5 to 1 Serving

Serving sizes are approximate. In the Un-Diet when you eat and what type of food you eat is far more important than how much.

Morning

Carbohydrates: It has typically been six to twelve hours since your BBG was fueled, and you still have an entire day ahead of you. Therefore, you need a significant amount of energy- and nutrient-rich foods. God made energy and the most significant amount of nutrients to come from the foods in the carbohydrate category.

Proteins: Because the body has been at rest, there is not a significant need for proteins and vegetables, which God made as your "building and repair" foods.

Fats: High carbohydrates are always accompanied by a low amount of good fats.

Morning: High to Moderate Carbohydrates /
Low Proteins / Low Fats

Afternoon

Carbohydrates: There is now less day ahead of your BBG, and some carbohydrates are still in the system from the morning meal. As a result, there is less need for energy so less need for carbohydrates.

Protein: Because the body has been used to a moderate degree, God created you to add a moderate amount of protein and vegetables at this time.

Fats: Moderate proteins and carbohydrates together are accompanied by low to moderate good fats.

Afternoon: Moderate to Low Carbohydrates / Low to
Moderate Proteins / Low to Moderate Fats

Evening

Carbohydrates: During sleep, there is not a need for "energy foods," so the body was not built with the intention of consuming high carbohydrate foods during this time.

Proteins: There has now been an entire day of body use, so God designed the body to require rebuilding and repair proteins in the evening. Additionally, your BBG will be moving into sleep mode. Sleep is the time when you were created to accomplish most of your rebuilding and repair.

Fats: A high-protein, low-carbohydrate meal can be accompanied by moderate to larger amounts of fats.

> **Evening:** Low to Zero Carbohydrates / Moderate to
> High Proteins / Moderate Fats

The Un-Diet Food Guide

CARBOHYDRATE GUIDE:

TIME: A.M.		MIDDAY		P.M.
LEVELS: HIGH —— H-MODERATE —— MODERATE —— M-LOW —— LOW				

PROTEIN GUIDE:

TIME: A.M.		MIDDAY		P.M.
LEVELS: LOW —— L- MODERATE —— MODERATE —— M-HIGH —— HIGH				

FAT GUIDE:

TIME: A.M.		MIDDAY		P.M.
LEVELS: LOW —— L-MODERATE —— M-HIGH —— M-HIGH——				

7 | THE BODY BY GOD UN-DIET

The Right Foods, at the Right Times, in the Right Combinations

There are many different types of diet theories. Most of these theories war against and contradict each other as each claims to be king. Nonetheless, the brutal reality is that, clearly, none of them have worked. Diets cause a great deal of suffering, can be dangerous, and truly get you nowhere. In the end, you almost always end up exactly where you started. Or worse.

Most diets are painful because they advocate restricting the use of certain food categories and nutrients and/or the overuse of others. All diets are in some way, shape, or form doomed for failure. Rarely do they promote the type of balance of foods and nutrients the BBG *really* needs. Even if they do work, you are only lighter—not healthier. It is also difficult—if not impossible—to stick to any nutritional program that calls for immediate and drastic change, a large amount of restraint, a bunch of work, and eating only limited or even obscure food choices.

It's Not a Diet—It's an *Un-Diet!!!*

Nutrition is very controversial because it is not an exact science. People are like snowflakes: No two people, regardless of gender, race, creed, sign, color, or blood type, are exactly alike. This is what makes most diet theories myths—and their success stories legends.

Diet theories come from the outside, from man, and not from the inside, from God and your own BBG. Now that you understand what different food categories do inside your body and how God designed you to eat, you can see why and where certain diets work, and why and where certain others don't. You can then take the best from each and create the perfect fueling program for your own personal BBG. *That's what the Un-Diet is all about.*

Diets don't work, but the Un-Diet always works. The Un-Diet is using Food By God the way it was designed to be used—according to the Un-Diet Food Guide. It is not something you are either "on" or "off." There is no goal and no beginning or end. It is something you begin living and just keep living it. It is not something you will ever be perfect at following. You just try to eat better, more as God intended, and keep on getting better.

It is not your "low," "no," "free," or "reduced" anything. You don't count calories, fat grams, or weigh your food. The Un-Diet is about trying to add as many Foods by God as possible to your daily fueling at the best possible times of day as described in your Un-Diet Food Guide.

The Un-Diet works for all people, all wants, and all nutritionally related disease. When you are eating the right food (Food by God) at the right time (according to the Un-Diet Food Guide), the BBG knows how to take what it needs for good health and get rid of the rest. Good health includes getting rid of or avoiding the "highs": high weight, high body fat, high blood sugar, high cholesterol, high blood pressure, and high anxiety, as well as the "lows": low moods, low power, low blood sugar, and a low number of trips to the bathroom.

THREE SIMPLE STEPS TO PAINLESS UN-DIETING

The Un-Diet can be performed by anyone, with any goal, and with any level of discipline or food dependence. The steps are simple:

1. Begin adding Food by God.
2. Begin reducing Food by Man.
3. Follow the Food Guide.

Even if you cannot stand eating any Food by God and find yourself completely committed to Food by Man, you will see remarkable and what appear to be even miraculous results just by eating according to the Food Guide.

For example, if you just have to eat ice cream and cheesecake or other high-sugar, high-carbohydrate foods every day, then eat them at the time according to the Un-Diet Food Guide when the body can best use all those carbohydrates—in the morning.

If you must eat bread and mashed potatoes, eat them early to midday as the Food Guide recommends to give your body an opportunity to use them.

If you love pork and cheese, eat your cheese omelet, sausage, and bacon according to the Food Guide. Eat them in the evening, without carbohydrates.

The perfect Un-Diet is 80 to 90 percent Food by God, only 10 to 20 percent Food by Man, and eating those foods at the right time of day according to the Food Guide. However, while that may be ideal, it is often too difficult for most people to do at first. The great news is that if you apply any of the three steps to Un-Dieting, you will see marked improvement.

I have had people follow the Un-Diet exactly only two days a week and see results.

I have seen people commit to just one Food by God a meal and get better.

I have seen people not change a single thing they eat and see great changes just because they ate according to the Food Guide.

Diet should mean "better," which is my favorite word. Especially if you keep getting better.

Owner's Manual Un-Dieting Recap

The Body by God Un-Diet contains the foods God intended you to eat (Food by God) as well as at what time and in what combinations the foods should be eaten (according to the Un-Diet Food Guide).

The Body by God Un-Diet, in some version, will fit into all personal nutritional requirements. It's not your "low," "no," "free," or "reduced" anything. *The key to the Un-Diet:* Focus on adding good foods, not taking food away.

MORNING

High to Moderate Carbohydrates / Low Proteins / Low Fats

In the morning, the focus should be on the carbohydrate category. Carbohydrate foods are needed in the morning because your system is depleted of them, and you will need power for the coming day. It is the safest time to consume carbohydrates, because you will have an entire day to burn or utilize them, as long as you do not eat too many. Remember, consuming too many carbohydrates will actually give you *less* power, which is the reason to avoid bread, sugars, and cereals, or keep them to a single serving.

Carbohydrates are also the best source for high-quality, usable fiber, vitamins, and minerals. Because the right carbohydrates are Foods by God, they not only will give you power, they will be easily digested and therefore not rob you of power.

Eating a carbohydrate-focused meal with a small amount of protein and/or good fat will help to moderate the rise in blood sugar levels. Good morning fats are contained in flaxseed, flaxseed oil, walnuts, almonds, and almond butter.

If this becomes a protein meal, the best protein is one egg yolk with one to four egg whites.

If Following the Un-Diet Food Guide Rules Only

If you do nothing else but follow the Food Guide, the morning is the best time for bread, pastries, and pizza. All have an overwhelming amount of carbohydrates that require as much day as possible to burn.

Preferred Morning Foods

Fruit. Your best source of fiber, vitamins, and minerals in the morning is fruit. Fruit is one of God's perfect foods. It is best to consume fruit only in the morning, and it is best to eat fruit first. If a lot of other foods are already in the food processing system, the fruit will not pass through the digestive process effectively. Fruit sugars caught in the system have the potential to have a harmful, yeast-producing effect on body chemistry.

The best fruits include grapefruit, figs, tomatoes, avocados, plums, nectarines, apples, pears, pineapple, currants, oranges, tangerines, berries, and melons eaten by themselves without other fruits or foods.

Un-Diet Tip:
Eat fruit only in the morning, and only one to two pieces.

Unprocessed Whole Grains and Sweeteners. Oats, grits, cream of whole wheat, puffed brown rice, quinoa, cream of brown rice, and jasmine or basmati rice are all good examples of whole-grain breakfast foods. The less refined and chemically treated, the better. Oats are typically the easiest to obtain in their most unrefined form.

Sweeten and flavor these foods with almond butter (tastes just as good or better than peanut butter, and it is healthier), almond or rice milk, fruit, unrefined honey, or maple syrup and not with cow's milk, sugar, or butter. This allows this carbohydrate breakfast to be very user-friendly and relatively Food by Man–free.

Less-Preferred Morning Foods

Chemical-Free Refined Foods and Sweeteners. Breads and cereals are popular, easy morning foods. The problem with these products is that they are refined, man-made, and very concentrated carbohydrates. Typical refined products contain danger-ous additives, preservatives, sugars, and hydrogenated oils and are not made from whole grains.

It is important if you are going to eat refined foods for breakfast, like breads and cereals, that they not contain chemicals and preservatives and that they be made up of whole grains that still contain some fiber and nutrients. Sweeten or flavor with almond butter, fresh fruit juice, maple syrup, unrefined honey, or raw organic butter.

Best Choices

Foods made with oat, brown rice, buckwheat, spelt, or millet flour, live sprouted grains, and quinoa. Although these may sound foreign to you, they can all be found at local health food stores and bakeries and taste great.

Use Non-cow Milk

Use almond or rice milk instead of cow's milk.

Reduced-Carbohydrate / Higher-Protein Breakfast

This is also a good plan for someone who has trouble digesting fruits and grains, is significantly overweight, has other digestive troubles, or has blood-sugar difficulties. Cutting back the portion of carbohydrates and adding more quality protein and good fat will help to control blood-sugar fluctuation. Reducing carbohydrates in the morning is also a good idea if you took in too many carbohydrates the day or evening before.

It is important to consume the highest-quality protein source available in the morning. As proteins and carbohydrates do not digest well together, proteins should be eaten with only a small amount of carbohydrates. The morning is not a good time to start a food war in the body.

An egg is unrefined and the highest-level protein source available. Pork and pork products that are typically consumed during breakfast are heavily refined, toxic, and classic Food by Man, and are not recommended as the protein of choice.

Basic-producing, acid-reducing vegetables are good to eat with animal proteins. Therefore, an ideal protein breakfast would be a vegetable omelette using three to four egg whites and one egg yolk, without any or just a small amount of other food from the carbohydrate category. Cook the eggs using olive or coconut oil.

When you add a carbohydrate to a protein breakfast, make sure to use *only* one serving of the most complete grain possible. For example, one serving of oatmeal or one slice of whole-grain bread.

Morning Beverages

Water, Fresh-Squeezed Juices, Herb Tea, Almond Milk. The morning is an important time for high-quality liquids. As you have not had anything to drink for several hours, the body is dehydrated. When dehydrated, not only are liquids needed, but whatever you drink will be absorbed quickly into the tissues.

You do not want to bathe your organ cells in coffee, tea, and soda, but with a great source of fluids like water or fresh, unrefined, nonpasteurized fruit or vegetable juice. Fruit juice, like all fruits, should be consumed on as empty a stomach as possible.

It is important to drink two to four glasses of pure water throughout the morning. As the body is depleted of nutrients at this time, and thus geared up for heavy absorption, the morning is also a good time for a high-quality vitamin and mineral supplement.

Hot herbal tea or hot rice or almond milk is a good alternative to coffee or regular tea in the mornings.

Late-Morning Snacks

In the late morning, it is important to not add too many more carbohydrates. Try adding one piece of fruit, one more serving of whole grains, or changing away from carbohydrates to vegetables, or eggs and vegetables.

Condiments

Fats: Ground flaxseed, olive oil, coconut oil, walnuts, almonds, and almond butter.

Seasonings: Butter Buds (replacement food for butter), cinnamon, maple syrup, molasses, and honey.

Preferred Morning Carbohydrates Options

Option #1: one piece or serving of fruit or glass of freshly squeezed fruit juice. (Drink fresh juice only. Pasteurized juice has too much sugar, and its nutrients are damaged or destroyed during processing. If fresh fruit juice is not possible, cut pasteurized juice in half with water or cut it out all together.)

Later or Option #2: Hot whole grain cereal (oats, grits, cream of wheat, cream of rice, quinoa) or brown, basmati, or jasmine rice or rice cake. (You can mix these different grains together to create variety in your hot cereal or to find a way you like to eat it.)
- *Add:* Ground flaxseed for good fat, almond butter, or sliced almonds
- *Sweeten with:* Rice or almond milk, honey, and/or fruit if you did not eat fruit earlier in the morning
- *Condiments:* Butter Buds, cinnamon

Less-Preferred Options

Option #3: All-natural, no-chemical, whole-grain cereal that is sweetened with fruit, honey, or unsweetened with almond or rice milk
- *Add:* Ground flaxseed and/or sliced almonds

Option #4: All-natural, whole grain, chemical-free bread with almond butter or small amount of extra-virgin olive oil and 1 whole egg.

High Proteins / Low Carbohydrates Options

Option #5: 3– to 4–egg-white and 1–egg-yolk vegetable omelet; no additional carbohydrates.

Option #6: 3 to 4 egg whites and 1 egg yolk with 1 piece of whole grain bread, or 1 serving of Option #2 or #3.

Late-Morning Snack: 1 Piece of Fruit, 1 serving of oats, vegetables, or vegetable omelet.

A Perfect Way to Combine Your Morning Options

- Eat fruit or drink fresh fruit juice first and then, later in the morning, choose from Options #1–4.

- Follow good food combining rules by eating a carbohydrate and good fat only at breakfast (e.g., oatmeal, banana, ground flaxseed, and almond butter) then two to four hours later eat a protein (1-yolk/2– to 4–egg omelets).

- If time or convenience is an issue, choose #2 to 4 and keep a piece of fruit with you for a snack later. Oatmeal and rice can also be saved and brought with you in air-tight containers.

MIDDAY

Moderate to Low Carbohydrates / Moderate Proteins / Low to Moderate Fats

The key to a balanced diet is recognizing the fact that not all meals are created equal. For instance, in the morning, carbohydrates were important to replenish your power stores to face the long day ahead. Now, as the afternoon approaches, lunch is a different matter. You don't need as many carbohydrates in the afternoon and most likely have sugar in your blood left over from your morning meal. There is now less day left, and so therefore less sugar you need to burn.

Additionally, you have now used your body to some degree. Therefore, you do not just need power foods; you need some food for healing and repair. You now need some protein.

If you have a physically demanding job or exercise later in the day, you will need to eat some extra carbohydrates at midday or in the early evening to provide yourself with the extra power boost.

If you have an increased need to lose weight, blood pressure, or cholesterol points, reduce carbohydrates at midday as you do in the evening.

Where breakfast was a carbohydrate-focused meal with little or no protein, lunch is going to contain moderate to low amounts of carbohydrates and moderate to high amounts of protein.

Morning was time for fruit, one of God's perfect foods. Afternoon and evening are times for God's other perfect food, vegetables. Lots of them.

If Following the Un-Diet Food Guide Rules Only

Because of their high carbohydrate content, try to get breads and pastas out of the way at lunch. As in the A.M., continue to avoid heavy doses of protein like red meat or large servings of chicken or fish.

Preferred Midday Carbohydrates

The best midday carbohydrates are going to be medium- to small-sized portions of those foods that look the way they did when they were still in the ground. The best lunchtime carbohydrate foods are starchy carbohydrates (sweet potatoes, potatoes, corn, peas, squash) and beans. Next on the list would be brown, basmati, or jasmine rice or other whole grains.

Less-Preferred Midday Carbohydrates

The next-best choice for carbohydrates at midday are chemical-free, whole grain breads and pastas. While still somewhat refined and high in carbohydrates, they have nutritional value and are not as refined as white bread, white pasta, and wheat bread that contains additives.

Totally refined carbohydrate foods like pasta, bread, and white rice cannot be properly digested and have a lot of carbohydrates per serving. These will be more likely to sit in your intestine, cause a spike and dip in your blood sugar, and make you tired in the afternoon.

List of Best Whole Grains*

- Whole rice: brown, jasmine, basmati, and rice cakes
- Whole-grain breads: live-sprouted grains such as millet, spelt, rye, brown rice, buckwheat, soy, and gluten-free
- Whole-grain pasta: rice, corn, spelt, and wheat

  *See Whole Grain Rule (page 68)

Preferred Midday Fats

Use olive oil, ground flaxseed, flaxseed oil, and avocado with your midday carbohydrates as your source of healthy fats and to control blood sugar changes.

Preferred Midday Proteins

Light Proteins. Because proteins do not combine well with carbohydrates and are difficult to break down and eliminate, midday proteins should be light, lean, and in medium portions. 3 to 4 egg whites with 1 egg yolk, 4 ounces of tuna, fish, chicken breast, or turkey breast are good examples.

Non-Animal Proteins. Beans contain carbohydrates and proteins and combine well with whole grains as an extremely healthy, non-animal protein lunch with only slightly more than moderate levels of carbohydrates. *Good non-animal protein sources include:* lentils, lima beans, and unprocessed soybeans.

Heavier Protein, Low Carbohydrates. If you eat a larger portion (6–10 ounces or more) of an animal product or a heavier protein, eat it with a salad and vegetables and very little or no dense carbohydrates like breads, pasta, rice, or starchy vegetables.

Meal Splitting

A great idea for getting the carbohydrates and protein you need during the midday without causing problems by combining too much of the two together is to split up these afternoon meals.

Eat a heavier carbohydrate meal first. Then, two to three hours later, eat a protein meal or protein then carbohydrates. This is known as "meal splitting."

Meal splitting works particularly well if you have a physically demanding job or compete in athletics later in the day. You can have a typical medium-protein, medium-carbohydrate lunch so as not to combine too much of the two and then, two to three hours later, add some more good carbohydrates to give you a power boost when you need it later in the day.

Condiments

Condiments and spices are good for flavoring natural foods. Limit fat use when consuming heavy to moderate amounts of carbohydrates. It is important at midday meals to use only moderate amounts of healthy fats and to limit or eliminate altogether animal fats found in dairy products and high-fat meats like red meat, dark-meat chicken, dark-meat turkey, and pork.

Use olive oil for cooking and olive oil and lemon for dressings. Flavor using hot sauces, tamari, mustards, and other condiments that contain no chemicals, bad fats, or sugars.

Good seasonings include basil, curry, dill, garlic, ginger, horseradish, mint, miso, mustard, paprika, parsley, rosemary, soy, tamari, tarragon, and thyme.

Late-Afternoon / Early-Evening Snacks

In the late afternoon, your snacks should consist of medium carbohydrates, or vegetables with protein.

Raw and roasted nuts and seeds are a great afternoon or early-evening snack. Walnuts contain omega-3 fats, and almonds are in the basic system producing, acid-reducing food category, so are the most recommended along with raw pumpkin and sunflower seeds. Soaking raw nuts and seeds for several hours makes them more palatable and easier to digest.

Another good snack at this time is vegetables with only a light protein.

*Nuts and seeds should be limited unless following the Un-Diet rule of only vegetables and proteins for dinner. Nuts and seeds are high in fat and so should not be combined with carbohydrates or proteins. See "Combining Fats with Carbohydrates and Proteins" on page 74.

Midday Beverages

Beverages consumed toward the middle of your day should consist of only pure water, fresh vegetable juices, or herbal teas that are unsweetened or lightly sweetened with rice milk, almond milk, or honey.

Preferred Midday Options

Option #1: Medium to small amount of starchy carbohydrates such as sweet potatoes, peas, squash, or potatoes with vegetables, salads, and light protein: eggs, tuna, or small portion of fish, turkey, or chicken breast.

Option #2: Brown, basmati, or jasmine rice.

Less Preferred Midday Options:

Option #3: Whole grain pasta or additive-free whole-grain bread with light protein.

Option #4: Vegetarian: Brown, basmati, or jasmine rice or whole-grain pasta or additive-free whole-grain bread with beans.

Option #5: Low Carbohydrate: Vegetables, salad, and larger amount of good protein (eggs, chicken, turkey, or fish).

> Remember that you can always split protein and carbohydrates into two meals. For example: Vegetable, salad, and tuna at noon, and then a sweet potato at 2:00 P.M.—or the other way around.

EVENING

Low Carbohydrates / High Proteins / Moderate to High Fats

When you go to sleep at night, your body begins its natural repair process as you rest. Protein is used for building and repair. So the best time for concentrated animal protein is at night, because sleeping is also the best time for building and repair.

In the evening, you must be careful to avoid concentrated carbohydrates, either altogether or as much as possible. Not long after dinner you are typically going to go to bed. Therefore, you don't want to eat a lot of carbohydrates and go right to bed because all that sugar power will not be used. *Try to stick to protein and vegetables only.*

The other reason to "just say no" to concentrated carbohydrates at night is that this is a heavy protein meal. A lot of protein and carbohydrates mixed together will wreak havoc on your fuel-processing system all night long, making it hard to sleep and even harder to get up.

If Following the Un-Diet Food Guide Rules Only

Red meat, pork, and cheese eaters would do best to eat these foods only at night and without any carbohydrates other than vegetables and salads. Avoid bread, pasta, potatoes, and rice with these foods as there is not much use for carbohydrates at night, and high-protein, high-fat items like these do not combine well with carbohydrates.

Preferred Evening Foods

Just Animal Protein and Vegetables. High-quality, lean animal proteins including fish, chicken breast, and turkey breast are your best protein choices. All animal products come with problems inherent with their use. As a result, protein choices should be extremely varied throughout the week.

Again, due to their ability to help balance out the acidic effect of animal proteins, their high vitamin and mineral content, and the fact that they do not contain many carbohydrates, vegetables should be eaten with the evening meal.

Less-Preferred Evening Foods

If carbohydrates other than vegetables are eaten in the evening, avoid the overly dense, refined varieties like breads and pastas and stick to the more moderate, natural ones like starchy carbohydrates (peas, corn, sweet potatoes, potatoes) and whole-grain rice.

Good Evening Protein

Chicken breast, turkey breast, tuna, grouper, mahimahi, sardines, mackerel, halibut, cod, rainbow trout, swordfish, sturgeon, whitefish, and lean beef.

Vary all animal intake due to toxicity. Free-range, organic, grass-, and/or vegetable-fed beef, chicken, and eggs are less toxic and have good fats, so are recommended if you can afford them, find them, or raise them on your own.

Evening Snacks

Snacks during the late evening should consist of low- to zero-carbohydrate foods such as raw nuts and seeds, vegetables, and animal proteins.

Evening Beverages

Beverages consumed toward the end of your day should consist of only pure water and fresh vegetable juices.

Condiments

Use extra-virgin olive oil for cooking and olive oil and lemon for dressings. Flavor using hot sauces, tamari, mustards, and other condiments that contain no chemicals, bad fats, or sugars. Good seasonings include basil, curry, dill, garlic, ginger, horseradish, mint, miso, mustard, paprika, parsley, rosemary, soy, tamari, tarragon, and thyme.

Preferred Evening Options

Option #1: Full serving of fish, turkey, chicken, or lean beef with *large servings* of vegetables and salad.

Less-Preferred Evening Options

Option #2: Fish, turkey, or chicken with vegetables and small serving of starchy carbohydrate or brown, basmati, or jasmine rice.

Option #3: *Vegetarian:* Small serving of brown, basmati, or jasmine rice with beans and vegetables.

Evening Snacks: Vegetables and/or more protein (low carbohydrates).

SPECIAL CONSIDERATIONS

More Power

People who burn a lot of power, such as an athlete or someone with a physically demanding occupation, may need to consume more foods from the carbohydrate category during the day. Because the body can effectively absorb only so much at one time, meal splitting is the best way to add more power foods. Adding an additional carbohydrate meal in the late morning and late afternoon is the ideal way to give the BBG more power.

For those who participate in highly intensive workouts or sports, it is ideal to consume carbohydrates directly after their activity.

The digestive system is the number one user of power. Unless you are participating in activities that burn up a lot of carbohydrates, more power is found by eating more correctly—not by eating more food.

More Muscle

If you have the need or desire to build more muscle and strength, you may need to add more protein and carbohydrates. This is helpful because protein is muscle-*building,* and carbohydrates are muscle-*sparing.* Meal splitting is important for adding more protein as only so much protein can be effectively absorbed at each sitting. Some good times for adding protein and carbohydrates are:

- *Late Morning:* Protein meal
- *Late Afternoon:* Protein/carbohydrates
- *After Dinner:* Protein

Children

The proper feeding of a child is incredibly important as their BBG is completely being created by what they are eating. Sadly enough, the tendency is for children to eat more junk, refined foods, and sugars than adults. This disrupts God's intent for their once perfect little bodies and has a deleterious effect on their future.

While they may burn up much of the excess sugars, chemicals, and additives found in these foods, ultimately they are not getting away with anything. In the end, the "kid diet" will cause symptoms of illness as their little bodies react to being poisoned. Many cases of common childhood health problems such as infections, allergies, adenoid problems, tonsillitis, overactive behavior, and learning disorders can be attributed to the improper fueling of children.

Kids need Food by God perhaps more than anybody else does. Making the body out of Foods by Man instead of those Foods by God recommended in the BBG Un-Diet not only will affect children's health but will limit their entire life potential.

TRICKS ARE FOR KIDS:

Tips for Helping Kids Live with the Body by God Un-Diet

The majority of things your BBG will suffer with or die from begin developing when you are still a child. What most kids are eating is less safe and nutritious than the wrapper it came in.

The standard childhood fare consists largely of Food by Man. As a result, fat cells begin multiplying and cholesterol begins stationing itself in arteries, the digestive organs begin to clog and malfunction, and toxic residues begin to accumulate in their young and developing systems.

Because children can be tough to feed, the tendency is to feed them the easy stuff—the stuff they will more readily like and the stuff that's more easily prepared. It is a lot easier first thing in the morning to open a box of sugared cereal and pour some cow's milk on it—which you know your kids will love—than it is to take the time to boil some oatmeal and slice in apples that you know they may not want as much.

However, remember that sugared cereal shaped like some sort of cartoon character with green, blue, and orange marshmallows contains so much sugar and so many colorings, preservatives, and chemicals, it is amazing they even survive the morning. Never mind sit and learn in school. It would be safer and more nutritious to feed them the box.

Kids need as much or more Food by God than adults do, and not less. While they may not like it as much as the sugary, fried, greasy, and colorful alternatives, eventually they will not only *eat* good food, but they will *ask* for it. By feeding them more natural foods, they will become more accustomed to their tastes, and their addictions to salt and sugar will slowly diminish.

While parents often get concerned that their kids don't want nutritious foods and won't eat them, the reality is that kids will typically not allow themselves to starve.

There are a few "tricks" I use to begin helping kids understand how bad Food by Man is for them and why they should start eating Food by God.

When I explain food colorings to children, I let them know that the colors are made up of much the same stuff as crayons and markers! When they understand that drinking an orange soda or eating a blue lollipop is like drinking an orange crayon or eating a blue pen, they are much less likely to reach for them.

I also like to read them the labels on their foods and then show them how some garage products or home and office supplies are made up of the same types of additives and preservatives. This is a great way to show them that eating ice cream, cookies, and fast food is a lot like drinking turpentine, Drano, or eating pencil shavings!

Commercial juice is a common kid filler used by parental units everywhere. The problem is that unfresh juice is pasteurized and filled with a lot more sugar than fresh-squeezed. To make this liquid safer, it should be cut in half with water to dilute the sugar. If the water goes on the bottom, the juice tastes the same and the kids can't tell. (Just don't let them see you do it.)

To get children weaned off cow's milk and dairy products, take them out into a cow pasture and ask them if they would want to suck out of a cow udder. Chances are, very few of them would say, "Yes!"

Snacks can be purchased from the health food store. While these "treats" are still refined, they are not filled with a lot of chemicals and, unlike their more artificial counterparts, they do possess some nutritional benefit.

If children become accustomed to the BBG Un-Diet way, they will get used to the right kinds of foods and begin making better choices that will not only affect them for a lifetime, but actually *increase* their lifetimes.

Let your little ones know that Food by God is what God *wants* them to eat. They want to give their fish "fish food" and their dogs "dog food." Well, God wants to give them people food.

Food Sensitivities and Illnesses

Everyone is sensitive to certain types of foods. Most of the more intense sensitivities are to man-made foods. However, many of these sensitivities are to natural foods as well.

When you consume foods your digestive system is sensitive to or that cause a reaction in your immune system, you may suffer from a variety of symptoms and possibly even serious health problems. These foods may also be hindering your ability to recover from illness.

Because of the less-developed immune organs of their BBG defense systems and their less-experienced fuel-processing systems, children are especially prone to food sensitivities.

Many of the illnesses people suffer from every day that are commonly treated with drugs or surgery, or go untreated, are due to some of the nutritional choices those same people are making. While children's food sensitivities are more obvious, many of the adult BBG health conditions are also due to the foods or combination of foods they are eating.

Sugar, artificial sweeteners, dairy products, refined foods, chemicals, colorings, preservatives, fried foods, caffeine, meat, alcohol, and white flour from the common Food by Man list, and eggs, citrus, wheat, rye, soy, peanuts, corn, and strawberries are some of the more frequent unnatural and natural foods that cause BBG sensitivity reactions. Just as common are the sensitivities from poor food combining and improper food timing.

Rarely do Foods by God have to be avoided completely. Usually they need only to be moderated or eaten at the right times according to the Un-Diet Food Guide. It is typically the Food by Man sensitivities that have to be eliminated or used sparingly. If you notice feeling abnormal following eating any food, cut back on it or avoid it completely.

AN EXAMPLE

While sitting in a restaurant for breakfast, I once overheard a woman at the table next to me complaining to friends about the fact that her three-year-old little boy, who was sitting with them, suffered continuously with asthma and allergies. I immediately looked over to see what her child was eating. As I had assumed, this poor little boy was consuming bacon, sausage, hash browns, and white toast with butter, and washing it down with a glass of cow's milk. For dessert, he knocked back some sort of prescription medication along with a spoonful of thick, purple liquid.

If the child was well before the meal, he certainly would not have been well after. This little boy was not sick; he was being poisoned. I wanted to let them know that he did not need his drugs; there were enough chemicals in his breakfast to medicate a large camel.

A banana or a bowl of oatmeal would have been this child's best medicine.

Many healing miracles will occur for people who adhere to the Un-Diet. But again, the Un-Diet won't heal you in and of itself. What it *can* do is remove the interference that stops your body from functioning normally and allow you to heal from within.

The greatest miracles that occur with people on the Un-Diet are the ones that you will never hear about. These are experienced by the people who *always* eat this way, and as a result never suffer in the first place.

8 | WEIGHT LOSS

How to Eat Like an Elephant . . . and Look Like a Gazelle

I was an amateur wrestler throughout junior high, high school, college, and for several years after college. I typically competed in a weight class that was fifteen or twenty pounds below my normal "walking around" weight. During wrestling season, I sometimes had to "make weight" two or three times per week. As a result, I lived in and out of a diet for nearly two decades. While making weight was often nothing less than pure torture, the good part was that wrestling turned out to be a weight-loss laboratory for me.

In junior high and high school, I was dieting in the dark. During those times, losing weight was extremely hard, and I endured a tremendous amount of pain and suffering. When you are that young, you want to eat like an elephant, but I had to look like a gazelle—lean, muscular, fast, and hard to pin down. It wasn't until after several years of college that I finally learned to eat properly. After learning what to eat and when to eat it, I was able to lose even more weight than before, lose it faster, and actually eat twice as much food.

The results of my wrestling laboratory experiments showed me that eating well doesn't mean deprivation. Today, I am able to eat more and weigh less. Now I can eat like an elephant . . . and look like a gazelle.

THE FIRST STEP

Turning away from Food by Man and toward Food by God is the first step to losing weight. A large part of being overweight is being poisoned and swollen from all the indigestible Food by Man stored as fat and fluids in your system.

Food by God does not leave fat and poisons lingering in the body. It is efficiently used, and then the unnecessary parts are tossed out. Not only does it *not* make you swollen or fat, but Food by God even helps to mobilize and excise some of what is left in the body from the not-so-desirable foods.

The Un-Diet (Food by God eaten according to the Un-Diet Food Guide) is how the Body by God was created to eat. If you follow the Un-Diet closely, you will begin to naturally move toward your ideal body weight. But if you want to speed things up a bit, here are a few tips.

The following choices will create the fastest changes:

- Do away with heavy carbohydrates such as bread, pasta, and other flour products.
- Do not eat any carbohydrate-rich foods after your midday meal. Eat only green vegetables as carbohydrates in the late afternoon and evening (as seen in the Un-Diet Food Guide).
- Drink more water and vegetable juices and less of any other beverages and cut out any stimulant drinks like coffee, soda, or tea.
- Massively limit—or abolish—Food by Man.

Owner's Manual Weight-Loss Warning and Recommendation

To avoid the failures that typically accompany restricting foods, just follow the BBG Un-Diet closely and add more movement (follow the Exercise by God program in Part 3). More movement allows you to burn extra fat and calories so that you may lose weight.

Start the Un-Diet plan, be patient, and move your BBG more often. This will not only speed up the weight-loss process, but it's also just plain good for you.

METABOLISM IS NO EXCUSE

The Laws of Thermodynamics and Poor Genetics Syndrome

One factor involved in what has become the overwhelming human weight challenge is something called *metabolism*. Your metabolism is how many calories your body is burning at rest or play. This process is basically determined by some hormone levels and the intensity at which the cells in your body are working and using up power in the form of calories.

A common misconception about metabolism is that some "lucky" people have high metabolism and some "unlucky" people have low metabolism. While those who are over their "ideal" weights often blame Poor Genetic Syndrome (PGS) for it and say they were just born with "bad glands," the reality is that the only glands involved here are usually the salivary glands.

While some BBG owners may have a genetic tendency to burn less caloric power and store more fat than others, in most cases the metabolism is caused to be slow or high by the individual. The belief that there are those that exist who eat like a bird but cannot seem to keep weight off is simply not true. There is something called the Law of Thermodynamics, which states: If a Body by God burns more calories than it consumes, it will lose weight; and if a Body by God consumes more calories than it burns, it will gain weight.

The truth behind metabolism is that the speed and efficiency at which your body burns fat and calories are determined more by the way you live your life and less by your genetics. Movement, multiple fuelings, and eating foods at the right time of day that were designed by God for the human digestive system all speed up or normalize the metabolism and cause the BBG to find or maintain its ideal ratio of loosely packed muscle to tightly packed muscle.

The Un-Diet guidelines, along with more movement, meet all the requirements for helping the Law of Thermodynamics work in your favor and maximizing your metabolic potential.

While choosing lean grandparents might be the most ideal way to burn the largest amount of fat and calories, ultimately you are never "stuck" with your body due to "bad luck" or PGS. If you have more loosely packed muscle than you should, chances are you were not born into it—but rather you invented it. The good news is that through God's Law of Thermodynamics and the Un-Diet, you can un-invent it.

Owner's Manual Tip

The key to altering or keeping your body weight where you would like it is learning to maximize your BBG's metabolism through movement and following the Un-Diet guidelines. While good genetics help, ultimately if you are overweight you have not been following the Law of Thermodynamics.

Overcoming Poor Genetics Syndrome (PGS)

Most of the people in my family are big and/or soft, and I have the same genetic tendency. Fortunately, by discovering the Un-Diet and committing to Exercise by God, I was able to overcome PGS by making different choices. I have been able to make these choices daily to get and keep myself very lean.

I have had patients complain that no matter how well they try to eat, they cannot seem to lose weight because of PGS. This, however, can never be true because it is against the law—the Law of Thermodynamics. In fact, when I walk past their cars in the parking lot I usually will discover the problem as I see the empty candy bar wrappers and colored sprinkles spread across the passenger seat that they did not write down in their diet journals. (I guess they didn't think it counted because they ate it in the car?)

Many of the people I have worked with who felt they suffered from PGS soon found out that while they had bad genetic tendencies, it could be overcome. For instance, one young couple who came to see me explained that both of them had come from families of "large people," and as a result felt this was why they were overweight. Ever since they had gotten married, the two of them had been putting on weight as a team. They felt that, due to PGS, they were destined to live a life of obesity, and were feeling hopeless to prevent it.

I told them how I had overcome my own similar family history, and it inspired them to begin trying some of the Un-Diet plan and start doing some more physical activities like riding their bikes and playing racquetball. Within sixty days of applying just a few of the Un-Diet principles and exercising just a couple of days per week, they came in for a visit and looked incredible. They got on the scale: He had lost sixty-three pounds, and she had lost over twenty!

Imagine if they had been applying the Owner's Manual!

DIET PRINCIPLES OF A SUMO WRESTLER

The sumo wrestlers of Japan are the best weight gainers in the world. Their sport relies on techniques that require massive leverage. To gain an advantage over their opponent, it is important to be able to apply as many pounds per square inch as possible. Therefore, the bigger they are, the better.

While some people are concerned with gaining weight, most people would like to lose an inch—or twelve. One way to gain a better understanding about *losing* weight is to learn everything there is to know about *gaining* weight. Nobody knows more about getting bigger than sumo wrestlers.

A Day in the Life of a Sumo

For the best results in your own weight loss efforts, it may help to learn everything you can about a day in the life of a sumo wrestler—and then do exactly the *opposite*.

A.M.
1. Wake up and eat.
2. Take a nap.
3. Practice sumo wrestling.

P.M.
1. Eat.
2. Sleep.

Sumo wrestlers rarely, if ever, vary their choice of food. The standard Sumo meal consists of large portions of oily meats combined with large portions of oily carbohydrates.

Six Weight-Gaining Secrets of the Sumo

1. Eat a lot of oily foods with carbohydrates.
2. Always sleep right after your meals.
3. Have as little activity in a day as possible.
4. Eat only two or three times per day.
5. Eat large portions at each meal.
6. Never vary your foods.

9 | RULES FOR BETTER FUELING

HOW TO MAKE THE CHANGE

When I originally began working with people to help them change their eating habits, the average person would fail miserably. The standard method of nutritional change is to take somebody's existing diet, throw it in the trash, and then hand them a completely new way of eating.

This method of "out with the old, in with the new" caused the average person who came to me to lose weight to instead gain eight pounds after only one session. Even cancer and diabetes patients would not follow my diet. They would rather die. No one to whom I ever gave a totally new diet for any reason ever stuck to it for more than a few days or a few weeks.

Following and sticking to a brand-new way of eating is extremely hard. In some cases, it is impossible. That is why I created the "Rules for Better Fueling" to help people get better at eating over time. As a result of the Rules for Better Fueling, I have achieved results with literally thousands of people who thought they would never be thin or healthy again or who had failed on numerous occasions to eat better.

To reverse this process of poor eating habits and move closer toward the BBG Un-Diet, use the following Rules for Better Fueling. These will lighten the burden of change and, in time, you will find yourself making better and better decisions and finally discover the health and the body you seek.

The Addition Rule

Positive eating is a gradual process. To be effective and long-lasting, change must come slowly, so as not to shock the system or the brain. The Addition Rule states that instead of eliminating the bad, you will add the good. So those of you who drink diet soda and eat a candy bar for breakfast every morning, you do not just stop that behavior and start eating nothing but fruit. If you do, you will only quit—or your brain will explode—whichever comes first.

What the Addition Rule has you do is add an apple to your cola and candy bar breakfast. With the Addition Rule, you do not take away; you *add*.

Most people are overfed but undernourished. There is no nourishment in their diets. Many modern diets literally contain no real food at all. It is all just fast food, junk food, quick food, and refined food, all of which are full of calories but devoid of nutrition. By adding healthy foods, you become not only fed, but nourished as well.

When you are told to "eliminate" something, it gives you an instant attachment to it and you only want it more. Noticeably, there is no "Rule of Elimination" anywhere in this Un-Diet. The idea of elimination tends to create negative thought patterns in the brain. The feeding system responds better to positiveness than it does to negativity. Eliminating negative food items from an unhealthy diet is a much more challenging task than simply adding positive things to the diet a little at a time.

Therefore, begin thinking positively and not negatively. To do so, call on the first rule of nutrition, the Addition Rule. Adding an apple does not do much to eliminate the ill effects of consuming other unhealthy foods. However, it does add a significant level of nutritional value to an otherwise entirely nutritionless meal.

Over time, the BBG will react so positively to these additions that it will begin to crave the healthier items as opposed to the unhealthy ones. Gradually, those nutritional items that were once merely additions could become the entire focus of the meal.

The Replacement Rule

The world is full of tempting treats that create a large amount of craving and satisfaction, but offer little nutrition. Traditional favorites such as pizza, ice cream, cookies, sodas, sugared cereal, fast food, and other unhealthy choices are literally addictions and create a real dilemma when trying to make proper decisions. To help avoid caving in to these cravings and addictions, the Un-Diet suggests an effective nutritional theory known as the Replacement Rule.

Many of the junk foods listed above, in their original forms, contain ingredients harmful to the BBG, such as preservatives, additives, MSG, and hydrogenated oils. However, today's modern health-food and grocery stores offer a variety of substitutes you can buy or make that are similar in form, satisfaction, and taste to these foods.

These substitutes come from Foods by God. They are all-natural and at least provide some actual nutrients.

Therefore, to phase out those unhealthy foods that leave BBG owners overfed but undernourished, follow the Food Replacement Rule and begin replacing them with more health-conscious substitutes. Replacing fat-, lethargy-, or disease-producing foods with healthful substitutes is an easy and effective way to start to slowly and less painfully change your habits.

Using this rule, you will soon find yourself more and more satisfied with the healthier substitutes to your cravings. Eventually, you may even be able to eliminate these cravings altogether. To help you, here is a handy list of common food cravings and their replacement foods.

REPLACEMENT FOODS	
Craving/Addiction	*Replacement Food*
Pizza: Store-bought or homemade	Whole-grain pizza with all-natural sauce and low-fat unrefined cheese
Ice cream	Nondairy, low-fat alternative (e.g., Rice Dream)
Sugary, refined cereal	One of the many health-food, whole-grain cereals with rice or almond milk

Craving/Addiction	Replacement Food
Sugar	Honey, fresh fruit juice, unrefined maple syrup, molasses, brown rice syrup
Salt, MSG	Healthy spices and condiments
Rich desserts	Whole-grain, nondairy, chemical- free, low-fat, or honey- or fruit-sweetened treats
Fast-food burger	Lean, homemade all-beef burger, lean turkey burger, or veggie burger
Cheese	Low fat, unrefined cheese and nondairy cheese-like rice cheese

The 10-Point Reduction Rule

On a scale of 1 to 10, if a craving is a 10, it will be hard to resist. On the other hand, if you can get the same craving down to a 7 or 8, you can control cravings some or most of the time. If you can get them down even farther, you can almost totally control them.

Therefore, the 10-Point Reduction Rule states that if you can reduce a food craving down below a level 10, you will have more power over your decisions to consume.

To achieve this elementary rule, it is prudent to start addressing those foods that currently cause a level-10 craving in the first place. For instance, a cup of coffee. This Food by Man beverage, which is loaded with the stimulant caffeine and typically accompanied by unhealthy dairy and sugar products, is a morning addiction shared by millions.

When coffee achievers wake up in the morning, their craving for this legal stimulant is a full 10 and seemingly impossible to resist. They crave the warmth, the smell, the taste, the sweetness of the sugar and cream, as well as the stimulating effect of the caffeine.

However, if, instead of coffee, they drank a cup of herbal tea with soy milk and honey, for example, this would mimic the flavor and warmth of the coffee. While this cup of herbal tea may not be as satisfying to someone as coffee, the similarity between the coffee and the tea brings the craving down from a 10 to a 7. They may still want the coffee, but the reduction in craving intensity allows them to skip the coffee many or most days.

The same can be done with a rich dessert. When the desire for an unhealthy sweet reaches a 10, you can eat a piece of fruit or something fat free or naturally sweetened and reduce the craving low enough to "just say no."

Everyone's Favorite: The Vacation Food Rule (You Don't Cave If You Crave)

Properly consuming healthy food as a way to keep the constant needs of the BBG feeding system satisfied is hard work. Beginning to eat people food is a slow process that often requires a significant life change to achieve success. In fact, it often takes years to undo poor eating habits. It stands to reason that if it took years to build poor eating habits, it will likewise take time to permanently change the wrong eating habits in favor of the right ones.

If eating well creates too much stress, it negates many of the positive benefits. The Vacation Food Rule was created as a way of making the process of change much less stressful.

Many people are either on a diet or off a diet. The Un-Diet, however, is not a diet at all. It is a way of eating that is something to work on for the rest of your life. No matter how satisfying your work, you need an occasional break. The Vacation Food Rule puts a food, a meal, or even a whole day of the less-than-ideal food choices in as a rule. The idea that "if you crave, you cave" is a myth. Rather than calling it "cheating" when you give in to a craving, occasionally eating poorly is actually part of the BBG Un-Diet plan.

While occasionally you will take a spontaneous vacation, the best vacations are planned. Therefore, suppose you are an ice cream lover. Well, if you eat ice cream every day, not only are you *not* on the healthy BBG Un-Diet, but you are going to get fat.

However, if you utilize the Vacation Food Rule, you set a short-term goal for when you *will* eat the ice cream. You may say, "I will eat ice cream only on Wednesdays and Sundays." Then, on Tuesday, when you pass your favorite ice cream parlor or somebody asks if you want to try their cone, you can resist your craving and say, "No thanks, I eat ice cream only on Wednesdays and Sundays."

Some cravings are so great, they are difficult to handle. By setting a short-term goal, you usually can push yourself over the hump and make it another day or two.

It is important to give yourself short vacations from always eating well. However, with the Vacation Food Rule, you may be able to drop some really bad habits entirely. What will eventually happen is that you will be able to put off some of your eating vices longer and longer until eventually you will be able to go completely without them.

Another positive side effect of this rule is that often when you isolate only certain days to eat some of your cravings, you will find that you do not feel well after eating them. You may discover that you have a food sensitivity to these vacation foods that you never knew about before when they were mixed in with other meals.

Eat bad once in a while, but do not quit the BBG Un-Diet. Crave, but don't *cave*. Take a short vacation once in a while, but then get back to work. Eventually, this rule will help you enjoy life even *without* the vacations.

The Food Dress-Up Rule

Initially, many of the healthier food choices may not seem very appealing. God-made foods tend to appear less tasty and fulfilling because of all the additives, sugars, salts, and fats that give less-healthy, man-made foods their flavor. The reality is that natural foods do possess good taste, but our taste buds have been dulled due to all the flavorings and spices in man-made food.

In order to make healthy food more palatable to your abused and desensitized taste buds, use the Food Dress-up Rule.

For instance, oatmeal is a healthy breakfast choice generally free of all the toxic foodstuffs that dilute and debilitate many other breakfast foods, such as cereals and donuts. The challenge is that oatmeal by itself does not contain much flavor, and preparing it with Food by Man like cow's milk, butter, and sugar will negate some of the positive benefits. Simply eating oatmeal and hot water every morning can become a real chore for most people. Even the most avid of oatmeal fans would become tired of just straight oatmeal and honey after a while. To make this nutritious breakfast more appetizing, simply prepare "cool oatmeal."

Cool oatmeal is your standard oatmeal with different *healthy* items added to dress it up. Adding fruits; soy, almond, or rice milk; nuts, cinnamon, granola, Butter Buds, or healthy cereals will dress up the oats and make them more attractive and fun to eat without causing too much mischief inside your body. Dressing up your healthy breakfast with nutritious food items is one way to avoid falling back into the coffee-and-donut mornings of your past life.

With this long-range goal of dressing up meals with healthy alternatives, proper nutrition can be achieved more realistically than by simply eliminating or giving up unhealthy foods altogether.

After a period of using God-made foods, eventually the sensation will return to your taste buds, and foods will require less dressing up.

The Stay-Full Rule

Food choices are triggered by something called "hunger." When hunger signals reach a high enough level, it will be almost impossible to make good decisions. That is why the Stay-Full Rule states that the way to achieve proper nutrition is not to get too hungry.

Consuming regular, healthy meals at appropriate times of the day achieves a proper balance of staying nourished while also staying satisfied. On the other hand, skipping meals and going hungry lead to a practice of becoming "starved" and create the need for eating anything within reach to satisfy the inevitable hunger pangs.

What is most satisfying and often most available are those heavily refined, fast, or fried foods that are full of fat. To avoid consuming such "junk" food, always stay full throughout the day with good, God food.

The Multiple-Feedings Rule

To achieve the Stay-Full Rule, it helps to also follow the Multiple-Feedings Rule. This last theory of proper nutrition states that smaller, lighter, more healthy meals should be eaten throughout the day to avoid the intense hunger associated with weight loss.

Most BBG owners have been taught to eat two or three relatively large meals a day. However, the body is better equipped to process small amounts of food every few hours. Large amounts of food cannot be handled well by the body and cause loss of energy, digestive dysfunction, and fat storage. Going long periods of time between meals also slows down the metabolism, making you even less likely to burn these large amounts of calories.

Multiple small- to medium-size feedings take less energy to digest, burn well, and speed up the metabolism. To achieve ultimate results with the Body by God Un-Diet and all the ways of better fueling, feed four to six times a day.

HOW I EAT

From Unhealthy to Un-Diet

My typical workday now starts with oatmeal. As a former sugar-cereal connoisseur, breakfast was one of the hardest things for me to change. I remember waking up and the first words out of my mouth were, "Oh, no, oatmeal!"

Now, I can honestly say that oatmeal and other hot grains are some of my favorite foods. I typically eat hot cereal one of three ways:

- Straight boiled oatmeal with a combination of ground and whole oats, ground flaxseed (a good omega-3 fat), sweetened with almond butter (a good basic pH fat) and half a banana, raisins, or honey.
- Jasmine rice or some other hot cereal like quinoa (a tasty, wholesome grain similar to cream of wheat, found in health food stores), or cream of wheat instead of or mixed in with oatmeal. I sweeten this with almond butter.
- Oatmeal or some other type of hot cereal cooked with low-fat granola, sliced almonds, and almond milk ("cool oatmeal"; see "Food Dress-Up Rule" page 114).
- Occasionally for breakfast, if I feel I need more protein, if I am cutting back on carbohydrates, or if I just want it, I will eat less hot cereal and eat a 3–4 egg omelet using only 1 egg yolk.

If I go out to breakfast, I order a broccoli-and-spinach omelet with only 1 egg yolk with no other carbohydrates or perhaps a bagel or a muffin as a treat for a vacation food. (See "Vacation Food Rule," page 113.)

Later in the morning when I am at the office, three or four hours after breakfast, I get hungry and eat either a piece of fruit, more hot whole-grain cereal, or rice cakes with almond butter. On nonwork days, I prefer to eat a piece of fruit first and oatmeal later.

At midday, I will eat a large amount of vegetables with jasmine (I love jasmine rice) or basmati rice, potatoes, sweet potatoes, or couscous. To add protein I add beans or egg whites with one yolk.

If I go out for lunch, I will eat a small amount of fish or chicken on a Caesar salad with steamed vegetables and a potato or sweet potato. Late afternoon, before going back to work seeing patients, I eat more of whatever carbohydrate I had at midday to fill me up for the afternoon and give me power. My preoffice power food is my last carbohydrate-rich food of the day.

Dropping carbohydrate-rich foods in the afternoon and evening was almost as hard as switching from Fruity Pebbles to oatmeal. I was used to coming home starving at night and relying on the bread, pasta, rice, and potatoes to fill me up and add flavor and variety to my food. This bad habit took a long time to shake.

The key for me was the Stay-Full and Multiple-Feedings Rules (see page 115). Since nuts and vegetables do not have many carbohydrates, I began to take them with me in the afternoon. This helped me avoid eating high-carbohydrate meals late in the day and allowed me to "stay full." When it came to dinner, since I was not that overly hungry, it was easier to pass on the carbohydrates and be satisfied with a piece of salmon, a salad, and some vegetables.

Once or twice a week I have a low-carbohydrate day. On those days I eat animal protein three or four times and cut out the rice or potatoes at my midday meal. On the other hand, once per week I eliminate animal proteins altogether, to give my body a chance to cleanse itself of the unclean nature of these foods and to take a break from eating a food God did not design my Body by God to eat on a regular basis.

When going out for dinner, I order fish or chicken and ask for a salad and tell the waiter or waitress to keep the potato or rice and give me extra vegetables in order to avoid eating carbohydrate-dense foods at night and poor food combining. (See the Un-Diet Food Guide on page 84.)

To meet my fat needs in the afternoon, I cook with extra-virgin olive oil and use it for dressings on my salads. In the late afternoon and early evening I use a combination of raw and roasted almonds, walnuts, cashews, and pumpkin seeds.

Because cooking food can destroy Nutrient Communion and kill the enzymes needed for digestion, I try to eat some raw foods like fruits, vegetables, nuts, and seeds every day. However, raw foods are hard for the system to break down, so that is why I will also add lightly steamed vegetables and roasted nuts and seeds.

My method of eating keeps me symptom free and loaded with a ridiculous amount of power. When I go off the Un-Diet, I can immediately tell. I will sometimes sense it for days. I will feel a little ill, have trouble focusing, look worse, have digestive and bowel changes, and feel a definite dip in power.

I do have some favorite Vacation Foods, and I take a break from eating healthy at certain times. On the weekend I will usually eat several not-so-ideal meals. Although, after years of living the Un-Diet, a lot of my vacation meals are made up of what many of my good meals used to be.

Typical Vacation Foods for me are food replacements like low-fat yogurt, cereal, and whole grain cookies, bread, and pasta. Once or twice a month or on a family trip I will really go on vacation and have a rich dessert or a heavy carbohydrate dinner.

Over time, I have been eating less and less of certain Vacation Foods, as the pain of eating pizza and Fruity Pebbles is becoming no longer worth the "pleasure." I also like to eat too much, and eating Food by God according to the Un-Diet Food Guide is the only way I can eat all I want and still look and feel like I want.

10 | CREATING YOUR OWN UN-DIET

SAMPLE MENUS WITH BETTER FUELING RULES

Example 1: Eating the way you have always eaten but *following the Un-Diet Food Guide for when to consume carbohydrates, proteins, and fats.*

Eat the foods you always eat, but eat them according to the Food Guide. Even though you are not eating ideal foods and you are eating too much fat at your morning and midday meals, because you are eating your carbohydrates and proteins the right way, you will see benefits. Over time, you can begin to add better and better foods and reduce the amount of fat in the morning and midday and see even more improvements.

- *Morning:* Donuts and coffee (High Carbohydrates)
- *Midday:* Chinese food with chicken (Moderate Carbohydrates, Moderate Protein, Moderate to High Fat)
- *Evening:* Steak, salad, and broccoli with cheese (Low Carbohydrates, High Protein)

Example 2: Following the Un-Diet Food Guide for when and how many carbohydrates, proteins, and fats to consume and use some of the Rules For Better Fueling.

In the morning, the ideal pattern would be to have a piece of fruit first and hot whole grain cereal with almonds, almond butter, or ground flax seeds two to three hours later.

If this is not possible, you can add fruit to hot whole-grain cereal or eat the hot whole-grain cereal without fruit and take a piece of fruit with you for a late morning snack.

- *Breakfast:* A piece of fruit (Addition Rule: Add fruit to your typical poor breakfast choices)
- *Two to three hours later:* (Food Dress-Up Rule) Oatmeal, honey, low-fat granola, ground flax seeds, Butter Buds (Replacement Food for butter). If fruit was not eaten first, add raisins or berries.
- *Beverage:* Hot herb tea with almond milk (Replacement Food or 10-Point Reduction Rule for coffee)

During the midday, if time allows, use meal splitting to get carbohydrates and proteins eaten separately (Multiple-Feeding Rule).

- *Lunch:* Broccoli, tomato, and spinach omelet (3–4 egg whites: 1 egg yolk; grease pan with extra virgin olive oil or coconut oil) with a small sweet potato
- *Afternoon:* Another small sweet potato with ground flaxseed and a leafy salad with extra-virgin olive oil, lemon, and/or vinegar for dressing
- *Late Afternoon/Early Evening:* Nut/seed mix: raw, soaked almonds, pumpkin seeds, sunflower seeds, and walnuts (Stay-Full Rule, Multiple-Feeding Rule)

At Nighttime, follow these guidelines:

- *Dinner:* Full serving (4–8 oz.) of salmon or mahimahi with grilled zucchini, green peppers, broccoli, and cauliflower
- *Late-Evening (Optional):* More vegetables and/or more fish, or a handful of nut/seed mix, and herb tea (Multiple-Feeding Rule)

Example 3: Eating the Un-Diet Foods by God while following the Un-Diet Food Guide.

- *Breakfast:* Whole-grain bagel with almond butter, one whole egg (Moderate to High Carbohydrates, Low Fat, Low Proteins)
- *Two to three hours later:* One piece of fruit

- *Noon:* Basmati rice and tuna salad mixed with one whole hard-boiled egg, shredded beets, carrots, cucumbers, greens, and extra-virgin olive oil or olive oil–based salad dressing. OR: Carbohydrate Vacation Food. (Moderate Carbohydrates, Moderate Proteins, Moderate to low Fat)
- *Late Afternoon:* Nut/Seed Mix or nothing if you used Vacation Food. (Low Carbohydrates)
- *Evening:* Sliced chicken breast stir-fried with extra-virgin olive oil, snap peas, mustard greens, cauliflower, zucchini, and broccoli. (Low Carbohydrates, High Proteins, Moderate to high Fat)

A Note About the Vacation Food Rule

During the week, you can add vacation foods or drinks to help you reduce the amount of certain foods you want to cut back on or to take a break from your standard menu.

Over the weekend, there are three suggested vacation mealtimes: One suggested vacation breakfast, one suggested vacation lunch, and one suggested vacation dinner. These are designed to help you set important goals of putting off the foods you crave the most until the weekend and add more variety.

If during the weekend you eat a richer or more refined Food by Man vacation food or meal, eat only two instead of three vacation meals that weekend. For example, only one vacation breakfast and one dessert after a meal.

Vacation meals can also be made up of healthy foods that are a break from the more traditional ways of the Un-Diet. Making your vacation meals out of healthy foods will most likely be more of a long-term than a short-term goal.

Example 4: Low Carbohydrates Days.

Many modern-day diseases and health conditions, including obesity, diabetes, high blood pressure, and heart disease can be partially associated with the presence of too many carbohydrates in the diet. Limiting the amount of carbohydrates taken in a couple of days per week by avoiding carbohydrate-dense foods at lunch or eating a protein-focused breakfast is a good way to accomplish this. Low-carbohydrate days or meals are especially good following entire days or meals that were high in carbohydrates, especially refined carbohydrates.

- *Breakfast:* 3- to 4-egg-white/1-yolk vegetable omelet and 1 piece of whole-grain, chemical-free bread with almond butter (High Protein, Low Carbohydrates, Moderate Fat)
- *Lunch:* Chicken breast/vegetable stir-fry and Caesar salad (High Proteins, Low Carbohydrates, Moderate Fat)
- *Afternoon/Early Evening:* Nut/seed mix (High Fat, Low Carbohydrates)
- *Dinner:* Mahimahi on a mixed green salad with olive oil and lemon dressing and a side of vegetables (*If you are a red-meat eater, dinner on a low-carbohydrate day is a good time to eat it.) (High Proteins, Low Carbohydrates, Moderate to high Fat)

Example 5: Vegetarian Days.

Due to the toxicity inherent with fueling regularly with animal products, it is good to give your BBG the occasional break by having a non-animal Vegetarian Day.

- *Breakfast:* Puffed rice cereal with almond milk, raisins, and flaxseed
- *Lunch:* Vegetable fajitas with whole-grain tortillas, roasted green and red peppers, onions, and soy cheese
- *Afternoon/Early Evening:* Celery with almond butter, nut/seed mix
- *Dinner:* Vegetarian chili, steamed broccoli, and mixed green and cucumber salad with olive oil and lemon
- *Late Evening:* Heated chocolate or vanilla soy milk

ANSWERS TO COMMON QUESTIONS

- Beans, peas, lentils, and unprocessed soy, combined with either whole-grains or nuts and seeds, result in a complete protein.
- "Soy products" (soy milk, soy supplements, etc.) are refined and thus no longer considered Food by God. Use only fresh soybeans or unprocessed soy flours to stay out of the Food by Man category.

- Almond milk and rice milk are good dairy replacement products. Almond milk has less carbohydrates and has some acid-reducing effects on the blood stream, so is preferable.
- Use all-natural spices and condiments without chemicals, MSG, or hydrolyzed vegetable protein.
- Use olive oil–based dressings and/or dressings that are low in fat and free of chemicals and sugars. Olive oil and lemon or a small amount of vinegar is the best salad or vegetable dressing choice.
- Never use artificial sweeteners (pink, yellow, or even blue packets).
- Never use artificial fats like those found in fat-free and reduced-fat packaged foods.
- Eat some raw foods (raw nuts, seeds, vegetables, fruit) every day because cooking kills the enzymes needed for digestion. However, vary the raw foods with lightly steamed vegetables and roasted or soaked nuts and seeds because raw foods take a lot of power to break down.
- All foods can be ruined through preparation (salt, oils, butters, dressings, overcooking, and unhealthy seasonings).
- Fish has good fat but must be limited due to the potential for mercury toxicity in waters. It is important to increase the amount of omega-3 Fats you are taking in each day. This can be done safely by taking four to six fish oil capsules a day.
- Eliminate or drastically reduce sugar, caffeine, alcohol, vinegar, salt, cocoa, artificial sweeteners, preservatives, and colorings as much as possible
- Never drink tap water. Always use some sort of water filtration. The best is either distilled water or water that has been passed through a reverse osmosis water filter.
- Fruit and fruit juice should be consumed only in the morning, but are still a better alternative to a rich dessert for something sweet after a meal.
- The best cooking oil is extra-virgin olive oil because it is the highest quality of olive oil and is monounsaturated so it will not break down during storage or at high temperatures. Extra-virgin coconut oil is also good for cooking because it is saturated, so it cannot break down either.
- Eat only processed foods that are made with "Food by God" and not those in which the nutrients have been removed (i.e., use corn, rice, or wheat pasta instead of white pasta and whole-grain breads instead of white bread).

- Don't be afraid to eat out. Today, there are few restaurants that do not have healthy suggestions on the menu or that won't specially prepare your food for you as close as possible to the Un-Diet guidelines.

BLUEPRINTING YOUR OWN UN-DIET

It is essential to your lasting success to consistently assess your health and how you look in the mirror in an effort to alter and tweak your Un-Diet to meet your exact needs. Because the Un-Diet is how you were programmed and developed to eat, most of the recommendations will work, but illness, sensitivities, and varying goals may cause you to change your fueling choices slightly.

Any Food by God you have been warned about using because it is "fattening" or has some sort of bad effect is typically bad only if you overeat it or eat it at the wrong times or in the wrong combinations. For example, some people are warned against eating fruit. But if they eat one or two pieces of fruit in the morning only, as recommended in the Body by God Un-Diet, they do not have any problems.

The Un-Diet Nutrient Evaluation Form will help you determine your reactions to certain food and help you build an Un-Diet plan blueprinted for your own BBG.

UN-DIET NUTRIENT EVALUATION FORM PROMPTS

Make copies of the forms (beginning on page 129) and fill them out for seven days.

1. Record the planned time of eating.
2. Record the actual time.
3. Record the planned food intake by category.
4. Record the actual food intake by category.
5. Record any planned or unplanned Food by Man.
6. Record why you ate: bored, tired, hungry, timing, business, emotion, social.
7. Record how you felt* right after eating.
8. Record how you felt one to two hours after eating.

*By recording how you felt after eating, you can begin to document food sensitivities. Note if there is a time of day when you are particularly stressed, tired, or in a lot of pain and attempt to pinpoint it to certain food choices or food combinations. Refer to common food sensitivities on pages 101–2.

THE BODY BY GOD 40-DAY PLAN—EATING FOR THREE . . .
1 PERCENT AT A TIME!

When I eat, I always try to remember that I am not just eating for me, I am eating also for God and my family. I am eating for three. With better eating, I know I can do more for them, and do more for them *longer.*

It is my sincere hope that at some point, you implement 100 percent of the BBG Un-Diet principles. Don't get me wrong, there are days when even I don't do 90 percent, or even 50 percent, of the Un-Diet. However, I always come right back to it.

Do not try to be perfect from day one. Remember, the Un-Diet has no goals and no beginning or end. It is not something you are on or off. It is something you live by just trying to do more of it, more of the time, until the end of time.

Follow the Body by God 40-Day plans in the Life by God section at the end of your *Owner's Manual* to learn the specific steps to eating 1 percent better a day for God for 40 days. Because the plan is about getting better and not becoming perfect, it doesn't end at 40 days. Afterward, you can continue to eat better for three for the rest of your long life . . . 1 percent at a time.

For more dramatic "overnight" results, see Body by God
"Overnight Success Plans" on page 349.

MORNING	BODY BY GOD UN-DIET	Nutrient Evaluation Form

Date	Real Time	Intended Time by God
2/24/03	7... (A.M.)/P.M.	6:30 ... (A.M.)/P.M.

Actual Food	Why You Ate/Drank?	Planned Food by God
Carbohydrate: Raisins, Oatmeal, Honey	Because it was time to eat, not necessarily because I was hungry	**Carbohydrate:** Fruit, Oatmeal, Honey
Protein: 1 Whole Egg		**Protein:** 1 Whole Egg
Fat: Egg Yolk		**Fat:** Crushed Flax seeds, Egg yolk
Liquid: 1 Glass of Water		**Liquid:** 2 Glasses of Water
Food by Man: Coffee, milk		**Food by Man:** None
How you felt after eating Good, but buzzed from coffee	**How you felt 1-2 hours later** Coming down off the coffee	

MIDDAY BODY BY GOD UN-DIET   Nutrient Evaluation Form

Date	Real Time	Intended Time by God
2/24/03	12 A.M./P.M.	12:30 A.M./P.M.

Actual Food	Why You Ate/Drank?	Planned Food by God
Carbohydrate: Jasmine rice, salad, broccoli	Very hungry (needed late morning snack) so I ate bread	**Carbohydrate:** Jasmine rice, salad, broccoli
Protein: 1 Can of Tuna		**Protein:** 1 Can of Tuna
Fat: Olive oil in dressing		**Fat:** Olive oil in dressing
Liquid: 1 Glass of Water		**Liquid:** 2 Glasses of Water
Food by Man: Iced Tea, Diet Coke, Bread, Sunflower oil in dressing (Bad Fat)		**Food by Man:** Iced Tea, Sunflower oil in dressing (Bad Fat)
How you felt after eating Light & Energetic	**How you felt 1-2 hours later** Nauseous from diet coke Fuzzy from all the caffeine	

EVENING | BODY BY GOD UN-DIET | Nutrient Evaluation Form

Date	Real Time	Intended Time by God
2/24/03	6:30 A.M. (P.M)	6:30 A.M. (P.M)

Actual Food	Why You Ate/Drank?	Planned Food by God
Carbohydrate: Salad, Zucchini	Hungry, just the right amount to make a sensible decision on what to eat	**Carbohydrate:** Salad, Zucchini
Protein: 1/2 Chicken breast/thigh		**Protein:** 1/2 Chicken breast/thigh
Fat: Avocado, Olive oil dressing		**Fat:** Avocado, Olive oil dressing
Liquid: 2 Glasses of Water		**Liquid:** 2 Glasses of Water
Food by Man: None		**Food by Man:** None
How you felt after eating Full but Light	**How you felt 1-2 hours later** Normal	

MORNING | BODY BY GOD UN-DIET | Nutrient Evaluation Form

Date	Real Time	Intended Time by God
....	.... A.M./P.M.	.... A.M./P.M.

Actual Food	Why You Ate/Drank?	Planned Food by God
Carbohydrate:		Carbohydrate:
Protein:		Protein:
Fat:		Fat:
Liquid:		Liquid:
Food by Man:		Food by Man:
How you felt after eating	How you felt 1-2 hours later	

MIDDAY BODY BY GOD UN-DIET Nutrient Evaluation Form

Date	Real Time	Intended Time by God
	.... A.M./P.M.	.... A.M./P.M.

Actual Food

Carbohydrate:

Protein:

Fat:

Liquid:

Food by Man:

How you felt after eating

Why You Ate/Drank?

How you felt 1-2 hours later

Planned Food by God

Carbohydrate:

Protein:

Fat:

Liquid:

Food by Man:

EVENING

BODY BY GOD UN-DIET

Nutrient Evaluation Form

Date	Real Time	Intended Time by God
....	.... A.M./P.M.	.... A.M./P.M.

Actual Food	Why You Ate/Drank?	Planned Food by God
Carbohydrate:		Carbohydrate:
Protein:		Protein:
Fat:		Fat:
Liquid:		Liquid:
Food by Man:		Food by Man:
How you felt after eating	How you felt 1-2 hours later	

PART THREE | MOVING YOUR BODY BY GOD

11 | THE LAWS OF MOVEMENT

God Wants You to Move
(That's Why He Didn't Create the Couch)

God built the body to move. All the vital parts that are presently keeping your Body by God alive, including your heart, lungs, spinal cord, muscles, arteries, etc., require that you move on a consistent basis. They need this in order for them to function properly or, in some cases, even function at *all*.

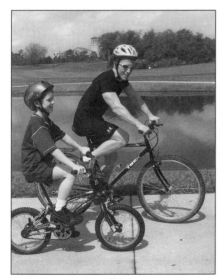

Dr. Ben Lerner and son, Skylar.

Regularly participating in sustained periods of movement, popularly known as "exercising," positively and healthfully affects all parts and processes of your Body by God. On the other hand, lack of movement leads to lack of survival. Keep reminding yourself that the body is by God, for God, and is God's, and the reality is, exercise may be the most important part of taking care of your BBG. Everyone eats, but other than using the muscles of mastication (chewing), most people do not use their muscles on a regular basis. While nutrition is important, how often you move your BBG is even *more* important than how often you eat.

In fact, with the added amount of preservatives, fat, additives, sugar, and other contaminants in our modern, processed Food by Man, physical fitness is even more essential than ever to avoid storing all that extra fat and eliminating all the sugar and poisons from the body.

If you are a "couch potato," i.e., one who rarely moves, your life is bound to run a little short. Inactivity causes you to live briefer, age faster, and grow larger. *That's why God didn't make couches.*

TURN YOUR FRUSTRATION INTO INSPIRATION

Put an End to Complacency

Intelligent people from every corner of the earth dream of health, vitality, beauty, peace, and a fairy-tale relationship. Tragically, somewhere, somehow, most of these dreams end up being shattered because of the inability to live in the manner necessary for them to come true.

Eventually, the frustration of failing to see any of their dreams come to pass causes people everywhere to begin dropping out of the race. As frustration causes enchantment to turn into disenchantment, most people finally just sit down and begin watching life and all the other runners pass them by.

Once they have given up, they begin to make dozens, if not hundreds, of excuses for why their troubled circumstances are justified. Rather than admit they have quit, they figure out a way to convince themselves that they are content right where they are. The ugly truth is, however, that they have not really become *content*, they have become *complacent*.

Right now, somewhere on the planet, complacency has caused someone not only to give up, but to accept defeat. Complacency has caused a countless number of people to begin living in a prison cell—and what's worse, they are okay with it. They are okay living a life that is somewhat less than full freedom . . . which is part slavery. *And no one is truly happy being a slave.*

Running the Race

Throughout my life, I have enjoyed the experience of running. I have always seen running as an opportunity to strengthen both my body and my resolve. At one point, after years of using running for health, prayer, or training purposes, I began dreaming of taking on the pinnacle of all runs, the marathon.

The problem with my marathon dream was that, out of the blue, I began to feel that the joints in my legs were deteriorating. Each time I went for even a two- or three-mile jog, I suffered severe knee, ankle, or hip pain. These problems eventually became so frustrating that I finally just quit running altogether.

Soon after quitting, I began to create several excuses to help me feel comfortable with my situation. I settled on the idea that twenty years of wrestling had given me bad wheels and I was not meant to run a marathon. I even decided that God never meant for people to run 26.2 miles anyway and that those who spent all that time running were wasting precious moments of their short lives.

While I still engaged in various forms of exercise, when it came to running, I was out of the race. I convinced myself that other forms of exercise were just as good and that I was content with my fitness program. Yet, the reality was I was not content, I was complacent. I had given up on a something I really loved and on a dream that I knew in my heart I really wanted to accomplish.

Fortunately for me, I began to see the iron bars I was placing around myself and, having seen them, I refused to be okay with them.

I refused to go quietly into that good night. I refused to give up and be complacent. I decided to see running a marathon as an opportunity to glorify God. I chose to see my desire to run as a desire that God had placed in my heart. I turned my frustration into inspiration and got back in the race for God.

I focused on the nutrition and running style necessary to bring optimum health and function to my joints. I also began to pray like crazy that I would finish the race and glorify God.

On race day, I made a decision that nothing would stop me from crossing that finish line because nothing can stop God. I told concerned family members that if one of my legs quit, I was going to pull it off, throw it over my shoulder, and God would help me carry it across the finish line.

I completed the marathon that day for God. I fulfilled a dream that He placed in my heart, and I have used many versions of this story to glorify God all around the world.

Taste the Freedom

At some point in our lives, we have heavenly dreams and lofty goals. Tragically, something happens between childhood and adulthood that sucks our brains right out of our bodies. Something occurs that turns a youthful, idealistic, uncompromising dreamer into an old, pessimistic, compromising realist. Some would say that what occurs is the reality of life. But what really occurs is frustration.

Frustration can lead to disenchantment, discouragement, and disappointment and cause you to quit and drop out of the race. However, frustration can also be the very fuel that drives you forward and inspires you to accept nothing short of victory.

The longer you have been sitting on the sidelines, the harder it will be to stand back up and start running again. Nevertheless, it is time that you became inspired not only to get back in the race, but to win it for God. Succeed for God, and you will make your dreams a reality, escape from your cell, and win back your freedom.

Once you have tasted freedom, you will never again be content being a slave. It's time to begin exercising.

> Although the Lord gives you the bread of adversity and the water of affliction [frustration], your teachers will be hidden no more; with your own eyes you will see them. Whether you turn to the right or to the left, your ears will hear a voice behind you, saying, "This is the way [Owner's Manual]; walk in it [get back in the race]." (Isa. 30:20–21)

THE AMAZING POWER OF MOVEMENT

One of the most *amazing* benefits of exercise is that from the moment you start, many of the health dysfunctions occurring inside your BBG due to being out of shape improve or return to normal. So if you exercise for ten minutes, then for ten minutes you are actually healthy. For some BBG owners that will be the only ten healthy minutes they have ever had. Isn't that *amazing!*

Some *Amazing* Benefits of Exercise by God

- Improves heart function
- Lowers blood pressure
- Reduces body fat
- Elevates bone mass
- Decreases total and LDL cholesterol ("bad cholesterol")
- Raises HDL cholesterol ("good cholesterol")
- Raises energy level
- Enhances and balances hormone production
- Aids in the sleeping process
- Increases stress tolerance
- Eliminates toxins
- Reduces depression
- Controls or prevents diabetes (blood sugar issues)
- Decreases the risk of injury to the muscles, joints, and spine

HEALTH AND HAPPINESS
(No Pain, No Pain)

For some people, exercise is an annual event. Similar to Christmas, once a year they break out their costumes and decorations, invite some friends over, and talk about getting together more often. Then it's over before they know it, and they put everything away until next year.

There are a variety of excuses and reasons that keep people from beginning or staying in a solid fitness program. They mostly fit into one of three categories:

1. Takes too much time
2. Too boring
3. Too painful

All these excuses should hopefully be dimmed by the Four Rules of Olympic Success—particularly Rule #4: "Inspired to win." The gospel (the good news) about the workout programs I am going to share with you in this section is that they are safe, fast, and effective. The aerobic section will show you how to get the most health and fat-burning benefits, in the shortest amount of time, with the least amount of effort. The Body by God aerobic motto is not "No pain, no gain"; it is "No pain, no pain."

The Body by God weight-lifting programs are done in as little as three minutes with a maximum of thirty minutes. These three- to thirty-minute workouts will give you many times the results you would get with hours of other types of workouts.

These aerobic and weight-lifting programs are challenging, but they give you energy instead of taking it away, and they help you recover from injury instead of causing it. (*The Time by God section at the end of your Owner's Manual will show you how to fit these programs into any schedule, as many days as you want, and with time to spare.*)

For true health and happiness, you need to find routines you like that fit into your busy day, and create results. Stress, even if from something that benefits you, like exercise, is still stress. If your fitness program causes you stress, takes too long, or doesn't give you a better, healthier body fast, you will never stick to it. That is why I have created routines that people are willing to perform on a consistent basis, that are extremely effective, and that many have learned to enjoy. Or for some, at least not *hate*.

Children playing for half an hour on the playground are having a good time while simultaneously getting thirty minutes of aerobic exercise and a leg and arm workout. They are happy, getting healthy, and while working out hard—they are not in pain. *No pain, no pain.*

European Vacation Inspiration

Europeans enjoy much slimmer waistlines, way less heart disease, and significantly longer lives than Americans. On my first trip to Europe as a United States World Wrestling Team physician, I soon discovered that more movement is one of the many reasons why.

I woke early my first morning in Europe so I could get in a run (a form of exercise) before attending the World Team practice. When I walked out of my hotel, I saw something that left me standing for a moment in a state of shock and amazement. The sidewalks and streets were unbelievably packed with people! There were thousands and thousands of people outside, literally creating a people jam. Having never been to a foreign country, my first thought was that there was a war and they were evacuating the city!

I ran back inside to ask the hotel clerk what was going on. She told me that most of the people in their city take public transportation to work, which creates the need to walk about one to two hours (or two to six miles) a day.

This type of regular, brisk walking every day is one reason for the superior health of the European people. Because rigorous exercise is part of their routine, they do not have to do intensive jogging, kick-aerobics, or watch steel-buns videos.

Back then, I used to perform hard, painful running sessions. When I was running and huffing, puffing and sweating, and dodging my way through the people traffic, more than one person looked at me, frowned, and muttered, "American." I felt like Forrest Gump.

Exercise Myths v. Laws of Movement Truths

Exercise Myth #1: Exercising hurts.
Laws of Movement Truth: Healthy movement is comfortable and can help to prevent, not *cause*, pain.

Exercise Myth #2: Exercise takes hours, and you have to work out every day to get or stay in shape.
Laws of Movement Truth: When done properly and at the right intensity, aerobic movement can be effective in as little as fifteen minutes, and resistance movement can be effective in as little as three minutes. Exercising the right way three to four days per week will notably improve your health and fitness levels.

Exercise Myth #3: Exercise can be performed only in a gym or with extensive home exercise equipment.
Laws of Movement Truth: Your home, neighborhood, backyard, and some simple dumbbell, hand, or leg weights are all you need for an effective, full-body movement routine to reduce body fat, improve the cardiovascular system, and tone and strengthen muscle.

Exercise Myth #4: Exercise is for young people, healthy people, or muscle-heads named Arnold or Rambette.

Laws of Movement Truth: A movement program is essential for every person. Not only can regular movement be performed at any age, it can even slow down or reverse some of the aging process.

Exercise Myth #5: Exercise is for people who want big muscles or want to look good in a Speedo or bikini.

Laws of Movement Truth: Movement is for survival.

THE LAW OF ADAPTATION . . . OR . . .
THE LAW OF "USE IT OR LOSE IT"

God put you here to survive. It is a rough world God created you to live in. Fortunately, God also structured the BBG with the capacity to develop survival strength through what is called the Law of Adaptation.

The Law of Adaptation states that, over time, the Body by God will *adapt* to the stress imposed on it by whatever environment it is in or whatever situations it is regularly encountering. For instance, desert cultures that are regularly exposed to the sun have adapted the dark skin pigmentation needed to more safely absorb the abundance of ultraviolet rays.

Similarly, in all parts of the world, the immune systems of the indigenous people have naturally adapted to deal with the local germs, their respiratory systems have adapted to the local altitude, and other parts of their bodies have adapted to the climate, the workload, and even the food of the region.

Part of the Law of Adaptation states that, as your body adapts to certain stresses, it further *un*-adapts to opposing stresses. For instance, people used to warm climates are not prepared for cold weather, while people in colder climates often cannot stand extreme heat. Likewise, people at lower altitudes have a great deal of trouble at high altitudes.

Due to the un-adaptation that is part and parcel of the Law of Adaptation, as individuals enter any totally new environment or different way of life, their bodies will often not be able handle the nutrition, the bacteria, the time zone, or anything else they are not used to dealing with on a regular basis.

For better or worse, your body will adapt to whatever forces you impose, or don't impose, upon it. In the case of exercise, if you participate in a regular fitness program, the forces you apply will cause you to adapt and get stronger, leaner, and healthier. If you rarely move, however, the lack of forces will cause you to adapt and get weaker, fatter, and sicker.

For that reason, part of the Law of Adaptation is: *"If you don't use it, you lose it."*

Adapting to Your Shape

Due to the Law of Adaptation, lifting heavy weights for short periods of time gives power lifters and farmers who toss hay bales, large, less flexible, round muscles. On the contrary, the Law of Adaptation causes those lifting moderate amounts of weight for longer periods of time to look more like an aerobics instructor or gymnast, with sleeker, leaner, more flexible muscles.

BBG Owner's Fitness Fact:
The Law of Adaptation and Reversed Aging

- People as old as one hundred can dramatically increase their strength, improve their balance, restore bone density, moderate diabetes, and diminish joint pain in just a few weeks of weight training.

- The minute you start sweating and your heart starts pounding, your arteries get more flexible and blood pressure is lowered. This lowers the risk of heart disease and stroke.

- For hours after exercise, your body is more sensitive to insulin, keeping your sugar levels in check and reducing your risk of diabetes.

- Being in shape causes your heart and blood vessels to work only a fraction as hard as they do if you are out of shape. A conditioned person will have a heart rate of approximately sixty beats/minute. An unconditioned person will have a heart rate of approximately eighty beats/minute. This means if you are out of shape, your heart will have to beat approximately thirty thousand more times per day than if you were in shape.

If you are a long-distance runner, your muscles, joints, heart, lungs, and various other organs and operating systems throughout your body adapt in a way to prepare you for slower, sustained movements. If you are a sprinter, your body parts adapt in a way that prepares you for explosive, quicker, short-distance running. The Law of Adaptation is why marathon runners have thin, long muscles and sprinters look like bodybuilders.

With the Law of Adaptation and performance always comes un-adaptation and altered performance. Marathon runners usually cannot lift heavy weights, and power lifters often cannot make it up a flight of stairs or run one mile without almost passing out!

Due to adapting and un-adapting, if a marathon runner were to start doing a lot of sprinting, he would begin to develop some shorter muscles designed for briefer periods of running. This would eventually inhibit his marathon performance. Similarly, if a sprinter or someone who competes in a sport that requires quick, explosive-type movements were to jog long distances regularly, she would eventually create a less quick, less explosive body.

Un-adapting and altered performance is the same reason a couch potato will eventually end up looking like . . . the couch.

GOD WANTS YOU TO EXERCISE

Early in my career, a fiery Southern woman came in to see me. She was somewhere between fifty and one hundred years old, about fifty pounds overweight, and suffering from numerous ailments. She was brought into my office by her daughter, who was extremely concerned about the woman's ever-failing health.

I gave her just a few small exercise recommendations to follow at home to get her muscles and joints moving and to cause her to burn a few extra calories. Unfortunately, this woman was very stubborn and set in her ways. She refused to follow even the tiniest of instructions I had given her and after a couple of months we had gotten absolutely nowhere in her care. One day when I again asked her if she had followed any of my advice she said, "This is the body the Lord gave me, and there is nothing anyone can do about it."

I thought about that for a few moments and answered, "Ma'am, God wants you to exercise." Something about that answer inspired her to obedience. She promised me she would try harder because this time she was going to do it for God.

I told her to begin by spending some time on a stationary bike every day at the lowest tension. She came back the next week and proclaimed that she was up to five on the bike now.

I said, "Wow, five minutes or five miles?"

To which she proudly stated, "No, five rotations!"

It wasn't much of a start, but over the course of the next few years, she got up to riding an actual bike one to two miles a day, lost nearly every ounce of that extra fifty pounds, and dropped several diagnoses.

She's much younger now, thanks to the Law of Adaptation.

MOVEMENT AND WEIGHT LOSS

Losing Weight the Wrong Way Only Means You Die Lighter

The purpose of weight loss is not only to weigh less, but to be healthier. Weight-reduction plans that use unhealthy foods, diet products, weird devices, drugs, supplements, or even herbal "speed" to help you lose weight may make you lighter, but not healthier. When people ask me what I think about these plans I always say the same thing: "Sure, you might lose weight. You will die ten years earlier, but at least you will be lighter." The reality is, about the only positive thing about losing weight the *wrong* way is that you will make it easier on your pallbearers.

The fact is, better health does not necessarily come by simply losing weight. To improve the function of the BBG operating systems, there must not only be less weight, but there must also be less *fat*. It is not only how much you weigh that causes you to develop disease, it is how much body fat you have compared to how much muscle you have.

The point of exercise is to increase the amount of real muscle and decrease the amount of loosely packed muscle, or what we call "fat." Having too little lean-muscle mass compared to body fat contributes to all sorts of conditions and diseases. High body-fat-to-muscle ratios negatively affect organ function, hormone balances, immune control, brain activity, and blood chemistry, and makes you more sensitive to potentially hazardous food elements like sugar and cholesterol.

Diet alone cannot increase muscle mass and decrease fat mass. Only diet combined with exercise will increase your muscle-to-body-fat ratio. This will not only cause you to weigh less, it will cause you to have better health. It will still make it easier on your pallbearers, but they will also have to wait a while before being called into action!

BBG Owner's Fat Caution—Fat vs. Muscle

- Fat has a tendency to produce more fat.
- Muscle has a tendency to produce more muscle.
- Fatty tissue is inefficient and burns few calories.
- Muscle tissue works more efficiently and burns more calories.
- Fat will make you tired and lazy.
- Muscle increases your energy.
- Fat gives you a poor self-image and decreased libido.
- Muscle enhances confidence and libido.
- Fat increases your risk of nearly all disease, as well as the need for larger dress sizes and bigger pants.
- Increased lean muscle mass will lower your risk of certain diseases and increase your risk of looking good in clothes.

BE CAREFUL WHERE YOU PUT YOUR FAT

Where you store your excess baggage (fat) has a lot to do with not only your clothing or hat size, but what type of health problems you may have.

BBG Owner's Guide to Exercise and Weight Control

Exercise Causes . . .

- A lowered set point (the body weight your body tends to want to maintain)
- Depressed appetite, particularly for negative food categories (most people will not follow a workout with French fries and ice cream)
- Increased basal metabolic rate (BMR)
- Increased lean-muscle-to-body-fat ratio
- Retention of lean body mass, which increases BMR
- Enhanced energy availability (to other organs and systems)

Fat in the abdominal area is fat that is being stored around the arteries and muscles of the heart. This makes someone with a big belly more prone to heart problems. Heart disease is the leading killer of both men and women, but one reason men are more prone to heart disease is that they are the ones who typically "get the gut."

Women, on the other hand, have a greater tendency to gain fat around the hips and thighs. While any body fat accumulation is unhealthy, the main issue with big hips and big thighs, from a woman's perspective, is that it makes them look fat.

EXERCISE BY GOD (EBG)

Born to Be a Survivor

In the beginning, God created man and woman to move. He gave them joints that bend, hands that grab, arms that swing, legs that run, feet that kick, and muscles that stretch, pull, and bench-press . . . *and He saw that this was good.*

Before the dawn of technology, everything having to do with survival required movement. Building shelter, traveling, growing food, and hunting for dinner all required physical action. Today, on the other hand, you can do just about everything without ever moving more than a finger. You can buy a house, make travel arrangements, and order lunch and never leave your desk . . . *and He saw that this was bad.*

I am always very leery about saying the word *exercise.* That word conjures up images of grueling long-distance runs, the latest aerobics craze, that piece of home fitness equipment that has since become an expensive towel rack, and working out in a gym with tattooed guys named Gunther. The reason these images are so unappealing to most people is that they are not the kind of movements God first had in mind.

Exercise should be safe, seem natural, and can even be fun. Just as with Food by God, "Exercise by God" (EBG) is the method of and intensity level at which God designed the body to exercise. When you perform EBG the way it is described here in your manual, you get fast results while avoiding or recovering from severe or lasting pain and not causing severe or lasting pain.

Exercise by Man

I was always an exercise overdoer. I spent the majority of my life participating in "collision sports" like football, wrestling, and rugby, and I loved to lift heavy weights and run hard. As a result of this penchant toward self-abuse, I have had to deal with pain and injury nearly all my life.

After enough suffering, I finally realized that God obviously did not intend for me to collide with other people, always push myself to my limit while running, constantly lift heavy weights in the gym, or perform many of the types of exercises I was doing.

What I was doing was not Exercise by *God*; it was Exercise by *Man*.

Exercise by Man includes: unnatural movements, strange exercise equipment, strange aerobic programs, abusive sports, and constantly pushing your heart, lungs, muscles, and joints to their maximum limits. These are all things that man, not God, decided were good things to do. Exercise by Man massively increases the potential for injury, organ failure, hating to exercise, quitting, or never even getting started in the first place.

For instance, the average "participation life span" of a runner is five years. After five years, some part of the lower extremities (a hip, knee, ankle, or foot) usually blows out. The five-year life-span number includes only those who are forced to stop running due to injury. This number would be significantly less than five years if it included those who quit because they simply don't like it. This is not because running is not an excellent, healthy, natural, and potentially fun form of movement. The problem is that these people did not run the way God intended the body to run.

When I work with top athletes, they are very focused on being physically ready for the next game, the next season, or the next Olympics. In order to do this, they consistently punish various parts of their bodies so they will be conditioned and ready to perform. While this may win a game, a medal, or a championship, it usually will not. If it does cause an athlete to win, it is typically not for long. Eventually, the people who always train to the extreme see a season, a career, or a life cut short due to a physical breakdown of whatever part or parts of their bodies they have been abusing or because of emotional burnout.

Exercise by God does not cause physical or emotional damage or destruction; it causes physical and emotional construction or reconstruction.

12 | EXERCISING WITH AIR

The Law of Adaptation and Aerobic Movement

One of the most important forms of movement is aerobic activity. *Aerobic* **does** not just mean a type of energetic dance performed to music while wearing spandex. *Aerobic* actually means "motion that requires the use of air/oxygen."

The BBG aerobic cycle kicks in approximately fifteen minutes into a sustained movement that is increasing your heart rate. These movements include such activities as going for a brisk walk, running, bicycling, mowing the grass (with a push mower, not a tractor), raking, skating, or swimming.

Aerobic exercise is also called "cardiovascular" exercise, or "cardio," because it conditions two of the most important muscles in the BBG: the heart and the lungs.

GETTING TO THE HEART (AND LUNGS)
OF THE MATTER

The Law of Adaptation has a profound and significant effect on the cardiovascular system. If you regularly perform aerobic (cardio) activities, every function needed for your BBG to move for longer periods of time gets better.

By regularly moving vigorously for more than fifteen minutes, all the organs, vessels and glands of the cardiovascular system adapt in a healthy way. They get stronger, more flexible, larger, smaller, or whatever is necessary to increase their efficiency.

The body's most important nutrient is oxygen. While you can go weeks without food (or at least *survive* for weeks) and days without water, you can go only a few minutes without oxygen. Through the Law of Adaptation, aerobic exercise, or exercise "with air," causes the body to take in and deal with oxygen more efficiently.

The BBG survives by sucking in oxygen through the lungs. Once the lungs have the oxygen, the heart and blood vessels pump it out to the rest of the organs. During aerobic activity, the body needs more oxygen than during inactivity, and it needs it faster than usual. Hence, when you do cardio-type movements, you cause the BBG to *adapt* by increasing the efficiency of the lungs, heart, and blood vessels to take in, deliver, absorb, and store oxygen. In essence, you become a highly efficient "oxygen-utilizing machine."

BBG Owner's Fat Burning Tip

For fat burning, regular aerobic movement is essential. It is during the BBG aerobic cycle that fat is utilized or burned.

BENEFITS OF AEROBIC MOVEMENT ON THE CARDIOVASCULAR SYSTEM DUE TO GOD'S "LAW OF ADAPTATION"

Cardiovascular exercise makes you a lean, mean, clean, oxygen machine. Some of the cardiovascular benefits you will experience include:

1. Better levels of oxygen in the body.
2. Better absorption of oxygen by the body.
3. Better lung function: expansion, deflation, and much more usable lung space.
4. More efficient removal of carbon monoxide waste from the body through the lungs.
5. More blood vessels being formed and existing blood vessels becoming enlarged and more flexible. The BBG *adapts* this way to increase the amount, speed, and efficiency of blood moving to and from the muscles and involved organs.

6. Improved carrying capacity of the blood vessels in order to better carry oxygen to the body and unwanted materials away from the body.

7. The heart's becoming larger and stronger to increase the amount of oxygen-carrying blood it sends to the body with each beat.

8. The heart rate slowing down because it is getting more blood to the body per beat.

9. Increased fat burning, which removes fat from blood and blood vessels.

10. Enlarged size, increased numbers, and improved flexibility of the blood vessels, as well as less fat and waste products in the blood vessels. This allows for improved circulation, decreased blood pressure, and less work for the heart to do.

REVERSE AEROBIC ADAPTATION—ARE YOU CHOKING YOURSELF TO DEATH?

Because the Law of Adaptation also works in reverse, a lack of aerobic exercise *decreases* the function and efficiency of the cardiovascular system. With less cardio exercise, there will be poorer lung function, less oxygen taken into the cells, and blood cells and organs with less ability to carry and absorb oxygen. There will also be higher levels of carbon monoxide waste in the body, less functional blood vessels, and a smaller, weaker heart that beats at a higher pressure and beats faster because it is pumping less blood per beat.

As a result of less aerobic activity, the BBG, which needs oxygen to survive, is less oxygenated; or, in other words, it is literally *choking to death*.

Signs of Oxygen Depletion

(Reverse Aerobic Adaptation—i.e., Choking to Death)

- Fatigue
- Injury
- Memory loss
- Joint and muscle pain
- Infection
- Sleep disorder
- Low blood sugar
- Depression
- Problems absorbing fat
- Decreased libido
- More difficult menstrual symptoms

BBG Owner's Symptom and Disease Warning

Many of the common symptoms and diseases people suffer from every day are due to bad lifestyles. This includes a lack of exercise.

Popular diseases such as adult-onset diabetes were never planned by God. He is probably up there saying, "Adult-onset diabetes? What's *that?*"

If you are hurting or ill, you must constantly ask yourself if you have created your own poor health reality. If the answer is yes, you must do whatever you can to begin building and creating a good health reality. Aerobic movement is a good start.

SETTING UP YOUR PROGRAM FOR AEROBIC EXERCISE BY GOD

Finding Your Aerobic "Moving Zones"

I have found that the major reason most people quit or simply *refuse* to move regularly for extended periods of time (aerobically exercise) is that it looks too painful, or past experience tells them that it truly *is* too painful. When you ask someone why they do not jog, walk, or bike to get healthier or lose weight, they will often tell you that they have a knee, hip, or foot injury, or some other sort of pain or problem.

Even experienced exercisers will often skip the cardiovascular portion of their exercise program because it just sounds as though it's going to hurt.

If it's not the pain that keeps people away from cardio, it's usually the boredom. Nonetheless, the truth is that if you do it correctly, you may really begin to enjoy it. If you stay in the right "Moving Zone," you will drastically minimize the discomfort of aerobic movement and practically eliminate your chances of causing or aggravating an injury. As a matter of fact, staying in the right zone is a great way to rehabilitate or recover from a joint problem.

Moving Zone workouts are blueprinted to fit your age, body, and fitness level by using your personal BBG heart rate. In order for Exercise by God to be considered aerobic/cardiovascular movement, your heart rate must increase for at least fifteen minutes. But if your heart rate increases *too* much or *too* fast, it can cause you to get tired quickly, release a ton of lactic acid into your blood stream, create pain in your muscles and joints, increase your chance of injury, and overstress your heart.

By controlling your heart rate and staying in the right Moving Zones during cardio-type exercises, you will burn fat more efficiently, reduce dehydration, hurt less, and enjoy more.

Zone #1: Maximum Heart Rate (MHR). Your maximum heart rate is the number of beats per minute your heart should *not* exceed during exercise. Training at or near your maximum heart rate is the type of painful, dangerous exercise people envision when they are making their excuses as to why they should not get off the couch.

The Fat-Burning Zones (Zones 2 and 3). Your fat-burning zones are the heart rates you want for experiencing exercise that is effective, pain-free, healthy, and as highly fat burning as possible.

Zone #2: Fat-Utilization Rate (FUR). The fat utilization rate is a comfortable way for anyone at any level to exercise and burn fat five to seven days a week.

Zone #3: Performance Enhancement Rate (PER). The performance enhancement rate is for enhancing athletic performance and making gains in both distance and speed while still burning fat. There is also some increase in calorie output at this level without getting into sugar burning.

Zone #4: Sugar-Utilization Rate (SUR). The sugar-utilization rate is at or near maximum heart rate. When you are working at your SUR, you begin burning sugar instead of fat for energy. At this level, there is high caloric output but also a great deal of dangerous stress being placed on the BBG joints and the cardiovascular system.

BBG Owner's SUR Warning

Training at this level should be greatly moderated and is typically for competitive athletes only. SUR exercising is anaerobic. During anaerobic exercise, your body forms lactic acid. This acid creates the burning joint and muscle pain often associated with cardio workouts. The anaerobic effects of SUR are why people are asked to consult their physician before exercising or to be "cautious" of aerobic activities.

Calculating Your Moving Zone Heart Rates

Maximum Heart Rate (MHR) = 220 − Your Age

Fat-Utilization Rate (FUR) = 55 to 75% MHR

Performance Enhancement Rate (PER) = 75 to 85% MHR

For Fat-Burning Rates (FUR and PER):

- Raise by 5 beats if you are regularly exercising.
- Raise by 10 beats if you are an experienced athlete.
- Lower by 5 beats if you are just starting out.
- Lower by 10 beats if you are on medication or recovering from injury or illness.

Sugar Utilization Rate (SUR): This equals 85 to 95% of your MHR.

Example Calculation for Determining Moving Zone Heart Rates

Age: 40

MHR: 220 – 40 = 180 BPM

Fat Burning Rates:

FUR = 55–75% OF 180 = 99 – 135 BPM

PER = 75–85% OF 180 = 135 – 153 BPM

SUR = 85–95% OF 180 = 153 – 171+ BPM

You can find your heartbeat simply by placing your fingers lightly but firmly over the inside of your wrist or on your neck just below the angle of your jaw. (*Caution:* Do not put too much pressure on the neck; this can slow down the heart, make you dizzy, make you pass out, and can be dangerous for anyone with potential blockages of blood vessels in the neck.) Another way to arrive at this number is to put your hand over your heart to count the number of beats or simply use a heart monitor.

FINDING "THE ZONE"

To achieve your Moving Zone, as you begin your form of sustained physical exertion, such as walking, jogging, biking, or swimming, find your heart rate in beats per minute. The best way to do this is to count your heartbeats (pulse) for ten seconds with a watch, then multiply this number by six to get your heartbeats per minute. Then, over the next five minutes, check it again, either increasing or decreasing your efforts until you have reached the desired Moving Zone. Check your heart rate every five to ten minutes to make sure you are staying in "the Zone." (A heart monitor can be worn to automatically calculate your heart rate for you.)

Caution: If you have any questions or concerns about your exercise program, your target heart rate, or if you feel ill in any way while performing exercise, consult your physician.

The Joy of the Zone

Again, the key to longevity is health and happiness. By staying in the correct Moving Zone, you should actually begin to *enjoy* exercise. Life is not a sprint; it's a marathon. Sprinting is a painful, gut-busting blur. The thought of huffing and puffing while slamming your feet and knees against the pavement will rarely turn any of us on for long. But if you can do EBG such as a slow to moderate jog, a brisk walk, or a steady bike ride while enjoying the scenery, meditating, praying, or even talking to a friend, you *can* stay in it for the long haul, breathe easy, and suddenly exercise won't seem so bad.

In fact, you may even learn to like it.

BBG Owner's Tip: A Great Way to Get Started

It has been found that aerobically moving two or three times in a day for ten minutes has many of the same benefits as exercising for a straight twenty to thirty minutes.

WASHING AWAY YOUR PAIN

When your heart rate goes up, your water levels go down. And vice versa. Whether you don't think you sweat or you sweat so much you can wring your socks out after just getting the mail, the reality is that when you exercise, you lose water. If you do not replace this water during your workouts, your heart is strained and your joints basically "get dry." (Remember from the Food by God section: "A dry joint is an unhappy joint.") Dry joints hurt and are very susceptible to injury.

By rehydrating yourself, you can literally "wash away" your pain. A good rule of thumb is to drink one liter of water per hour of aerobic exercise. Often, this means that you have to drink water while you are performing your aerobic task and not just before or after.

If performing aerobic movements outside, get used to doing it while carrying water in your hand, in a water bottle belt, or have water stashed somewhere along your route. As a general rule, drink at least one-half your body weight in ounces of water every day. Sip on water before, during, and after your exercise sessions. Since dehydration can elevate your heart rate and cause the readings of your heart rate to be much higher than expected, adequate hydration is essential.

It is a good idea to take in water constantly throughout the day, especially when heat or humidity could be a concern. Drink water slowly. Do not guzzle large amounts all at once before you are ready to exercise.

BBG Owner's Joint-Saving Advice

Check "Back to Basics" on page 76 in the Food by God section of your *Owner's Manual* to see how adding more basic-causing, acid-neutralizing foods like green vegetables, almonds, and good fats, in addition to water, will also help in the recovery and prevention of exercise-induced painful joints.

OLDER BUT SMARTER . . . OR . . . YOU CAN TEACH AN OLD DOG TO GO RUNNING

When I hit thirty, I found myself suffering from ex-jock disease. Years of hard-core sports and SUR workouts that pushed my joints past their limits had left me with a number of weaknesses. I began to have a new injury every month, and I was constantly eliminating certain exercises from my program because they hurt too much.

When I reached a point that I could not run for more than a couple of miles before my knees, ankles, and/or feet began to kill me, often leaving me limping around for days, I decided that I had to figure something out. Refusing to get old and still never having achieved my lifelong dream of running a marathon, I thought long and hard about what needed to be done to get my youthful wheels back. I came up with three problems:

1. I had to get rid of my macho need to run fast. I had to start training in the fat-burning zones and not in the acid-producing, sugar-burning zones.

2. I would work out or run for twenty to sixty minutes and not drink anything until afterward. Therefore, I needed to start keeping water with me when I exercised.

3. I had to eat more foods that reduced acid levels and created a more basic environment in my system. I needed to add more good fat to my diet and make an effort to take in more green leafy lettuces and green vegetables so I had a less-acidic blood stream.

When I started running in the right zone, started carrying water with me during my runs and workouts, and got *"back to basics"* with my nutrition, I felt the true measure of God's healing and forgiveness. My lower extremities healed, and I was able to realize a dream by finishing the Disney Marathon.

I finished an hour behind Minnie and Pluto, but I finished.

YOUR AEROBIC EBG ROUTINE

The safest, most efficient way to begin all cardiovascular activity is by moving very slowly. Start out your runs, walks, bike rides, swimming, etc., by warming up at a very slow pace. Finish your routine by cooling down the same way, at a very slow pace.

The BBG was built as a very efficient machine, designed to primarily burn fat for fuel. The key to maximizing the use of fat as fuel is to build your heart rate up to your targeted Moving Zone slowly and gradually. Following your slow pace warm-up, increase your speed little by little until you reach your Moving Zone, and then level off. By slowly and steadily bringing up your heart rate, you encourage your body to burn fat right from the beginning of your workout. In fact, the more gradually you bring your heart rate up, the richer in fat your fuel source will be.

During the cooldown phase of your moving session, you want your heart rate to slowly drop to your warm-up rate. Most people skip this portion of the workout, although it is potentially even more important than the warm-up. The cooldown helps your body transition from an active state into a more sedentary one. This lets your body redirect the flow of blood away from the large working muscles and back to the internal organs and brain.

Warm-up and cooldown periods should each last a minimum of five to ten minutes. If you have never been on a regular running program, you probably want to start by running for only a fifteen-minute period (not including warm-up and cooldown). If you desire to improve, you can increase the time you move by five to ten minutes as you get in better and better condition.

RUNNING POSTURE AND POSITION

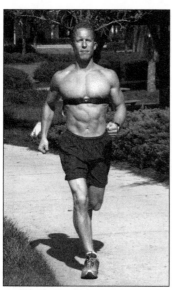
Dr. Ben Lerner

Running Picture Posture:

- Head and shoulders back.
- Back straight.
- Eyes facing straight forward.
- Arms stay bent at your sides.
- Breathe in through your nose and fill your stomach with air right behind your belly button. Breathe out slowly through mouth by expanding your chest.
- Feet gently roll from heel to toe.
- Don't work any harder than you have to, or work as hard as you can—it all depends on your goal.

Choose Your Rate Based on Your Goal

Goal #1: Fat-Utilization Rate (FUR) (Movement is at a comfortable, steady pace you enjoy.) FUR moves you into a moderate, aerobic, fat-burning state, which will safely help you lose fat and increase your overall health.

Goal #2: Performance-Enhancement Rate (PER) (Movement is at a swifter rate of speed that is sustainable.) PER has the objective of helping you increase your efficiency and learning to be more productive as you move. This rate will continue to burn fat for fuel while increasing performance times and efficiency.

PER is used in preparation for performing in events that require sustained movement. For instance, long-distance running, rugby, or soccer.

Goal #3: Sugar Utilization Rate (SUR) (Movement is up-tempo, challenging, and there is a limit to how long you can sustain the intensity.) SUR provides your body with the ability to perform at high intensity. Athletes who participate in sports that require quick bursts of movement, such as sprinting, wrestling, lifting, or jumping, will benefit from training in the SUR zone.

SUR training will increase performance in all activities as it enhances different components of energy output and heart, lung, and muscle function. Most sporting activities require a blend of fat-burning and sugar-burning abilities. Therefore, competitive athletes should blend all three levels of training into their workouts.

Combining FUR, PER, and SUR

To increase your heart rate and move from FUR to PER to SUR, you can perform the movement faster, at a steeper incline, or increase the weight or tension, depending on the form of exercise.

SAMPLE AEROBIC ROUTINES

To Set Up Your Personal Aerobic Program:

1. Calculate your Moving Zones.
2. Choose an exercise.
3. Begin the exercise with a five- to ten-minute warm-up.
4. Move through the exercise, increasing the speed, tension, or incline so you can achieve or stay in the right zone.
5. Finish the exercise with a five- to ten-minute cooldown.
6. Following the activity, write down what speed, tension, or incline was necessary to achieve the particular zone.

EXAMPLE AEROBIC ROUTINES

EXAMPLE 30-MINUTE CARDIOVASCULAR MOVEMENT
(+10 MINUTE WARM-UP/COOLDOWN= 40 MINUTE TOTAL)

FOR FAT BURNING

Name: _Rachel (beginner with knee injury)_

Age: _50_ Gender: _Female_

ACTIVITY: _Stationary BIKE_

FUR - Fat-Utilization Rate PER - Performance Enhancement Rate SUR - Sugar-Utilization Rate

FUR: _94-127 (-10)_ PER: _127-144 (-10)_ SUR: _144-161_

MOVING ZONE LEVELS			
TIME (Elapsed)	TIME (Per Stage)	HEART RATE	SPEED/INCLINE OR LEVEL/RPM	HEART RATE (Real)
0:00	0:00	Resting Heart Rate (RHR)+	0/0	RHR 75-80
5:00	5:00	Below - FUR	1/65	80-85
7:00	2:00	Near - FUR	1/75	85-90
9:00	2:00	Nearer - FUR	1/80	90-95
14:00	5:00	First 1% - FUR	2/80	95-100
19:00	5:00	First 10% - FUR	3/85	100-110
24:00	5:00	First 50% - FUR	4/85	110-115
29:00	5:00	First 10% - FUR	3/85	115-105
32:00	3:00	First 1% - FUR	2/75	105-95
35:00	3:00	Near - FUR	1/70	95-90
40:00	5:00	Below - FUR - RHR+	1/60-65	90-80

Example Aerobic Routines

EXAMPLE 40-MINUTE CARDIOVASCULAR MOVEMENT
(+10 MINUTE WARM-UP/COOLDOWN= 50 MINUTE TOTAL)

FOR FAT BURNING AND IMPROVED PERFORMANCE

Name: _Moses_

Age: _40_   Gender: _Male_

ACTIVITY: _Running_

WARNING - Before you begin: Never start an exercise program without first consulting your physician. Those with a personal history of heart disease, high blood pressure, high cholesterol, cancer, diabetes, or who smoke or are overweight should begin exercising with professional supervision.

FUR - Fat-Utilization Rate   **PER** - Performance Enhancement Rate   **SUR** - Sugar-Utilization Rate

FUR: _99-135_   PER: _135-153_   SUR: _153-171_

MOVING ZONE LEVELS	TIME (Elapsed)	TIME (Per Stage)	HEART RATE	SPEED	HEART RATE (Real)
	0:00	0:00	Resting Heart Rate (RHR)+	0/0 Mph	RHR 72-75
	5:00	5:00	Below - FUR	3-3.5 Mph	75-80
	7:00	2:00	Near - FUR	4-4.5 Mph	80-85
	9:00	2:00	Nearer - FUR	5 Mph	85-90
	11:00	2:00	First 1% - FUR	5-5.5 Mph	95-99
	13:00	2:00	First 10% - FUR	5.5 Mph	99-110
	15:00	2:00	First 10% - FUR	5.5 Mph	99-110
	18:00	3:00	First 50% - FUR	5.5 Mph	110-117
	21:00	3:00	Last 50% - FUR	6 Mph	117-135
	25:00	4:00	First 50% - PER	6 Mph	135-145
	29:00	4:00	First 50% - PER	6.5 Mph	135-145
	33:00	4:00	Last 50% - PER	6.5 Mph	145-153
	36:00	3:00	Last 50% - PER	6.5 Mph	153-145
	39:00	3:00	PER - FUR	6 Mph	145-135
	42:00	3:00	Last 50% - FUR	6 Mph	135-117
	45:00	3:00	First 50% - FUR	5.5 Mph	117-99
	50:00	5:00	First 10% - FUR - RHR +	5.5-3 Mph	99-75

EXAMPLE AEROBIC ROUTINES

40-MINUTE CARDIOVASCULAR MOVEMENT
(+10 MINUTE WARM-UP/COOLDOWN= 50 MINUTE TOTAL)

FOR FAT BURNING AND SPORTS/PEAK PERFORMANCE

Name: *Sampson (Experienced Runner?)*
Age: *40*   Gender: *Male*
ACTIVITY: *Running*

FUR - Fat-Utilization Rate   PER - Performance Enhancement Rate   SUR - Sugar-Utilization Rate

FUR: *99-135 (+10)*   PER: *135-153 (+10)*   SUR: *53-171*

MOVING ZONE LEVELS	TIME (Elapsed)	TIME (Per Stage)	HEART RATE	SPEED/INCLINE	HEART RATE (Real)
	0:00	0:00	Resting Heart Rate (RHR)+	Mph/0	RHR 72-75
	5:00	5:00	Below - FUR	3-3.5 Mph/ 0	75-80
	7:00	2:00	Near - FUR	4-5 Mph/ 0	80-85
	9:00	2:00	Nearer - FUR	5-5.5 Mph/ 1	85-95
	11:00	2:00	First 1% - FUR	5-5.6 Mph/ 2	95-110
	13:00	2:00	First 50% - FUR	6 Mph/ 2	110-120
	15:00	2:00	First 50% - FUR	6.5 Mph/ 3	120-140
	17:00	2:00	SUR	7.5-8.5 Mph/ 4	153-171
	19:00	2:00	PER - FUR	7-6 Mph/ 3-2	171-145
	21:00	2:00	PER	7 Mph/ 3	145-163
	24:00	3:00	SUR	8.5 Mph/ 4	163-171
	26:00	2:00	PER - FUR	7-6 Mph/ 3-2	171-145
	28:00	2:00	PER	7 Mph/ 3	145-163
	32:00	4:00	SUR	8.5 Mph/ 4	163-171
	34:00	2:00	PER - FUR	7-6 Mph/ 3-2	171-145
	36:00	2:00	PER	7 Mph/ 3	145-163
	41:00	5:00	SUR	8.5 Mph/ 4	163-171
	45:00	4:00	PER - FUR	7-6 Mph/ 3-2	171-127
	50:00	5:00	FUR - RHR+	5.5 Mph/ 3-0	127-72+

PERSONAL AEROBIC ROUTINES

30-MINUTE CARDIOVASCULAR MOVEMENT

(+10 MINUTE WARM-UP/COOLDOWN = 40 MINUTE TOTAL)

FOR FAT BURNING

Name: _____

Age: _____ Gender: _____

ACTIVITY:

FUR - Fat-Utilization Rate   PER - Performance Enhancement Rate   SUR - Sugar-Utilization Rate

FUR: _____   PER: _____   SUR: _____

MOVING ZONE LEVELS				
TIME (Elapsed)	TIME (Per Stage)	HEART RATE	SPEED/INCLINE OR LEVEL/RPM	HEART RATE (Real)
0:00	0:00	Resting Heart Rate (RHR)+	Mph/	RHR
5:00	5:00	Below - FUR	Mph/	
7:00	2:00	Near - FUR	Mph/	
9:00	2:00	Nearer - FUR	Mph/	
14:00	5:00	First 1% - FUR	Mph/	
19:00	5:00	First 10% - FUR	Mph/	
24:00	5:00	First 50% - FUR	Mph/	
29:00	5:00	First 10% - FUR	Mph/	
32:00	3:00	First 1% - FUR	Mph/	
35:00	3:00	Near - FUR	Mph/	
40:00	5:00	Below - FUR - RHR+	Mph/	

PERSONAL AEROBIC ROUTINES

40-Minute Cardiovascular Movement
(+10 minute Warm-Up/Cooldown= 50 minute Total)

FOR FAT BURNING AND IMPROVED PERFORMANCE

Name: _____

Age: _____ Gender: _____

ACTIVITY: _____

WARNING - Before you begin: Never start an exercise program without first consulting your physician. Those with a personal history of heart disease, high blood pressure, high cholesterol, cancer, diabetes, or who smoke or are overweight should begin exercising with professional supervision.

FUR - Fat-Utilization Rate   **PER** - Performance Enhancement Rate   **SUR** - Sugar-Utilization Rate

FUR: _____   PER: _____   SUR: _____

MOVING ZONE LEVELS	TIME (Elapsed)	TIME (Per Stage)	HEART RATE	SPEED/INCLINE OR LEVEL/RPM	HEART RATE (Real)
	0:00	0:00	Resting Heart Rate (RHR)+	0Mph/0	
	5:00	5:00	Below - FUR	Mph/	
	7:00	2:00	Near - FUR	Mph/	
	9:00	2:00	Nearer - FUR	Mph/	
	11:00	2:00	First 1% - FUR	Mph/	
	13:00	2:00	First 10% - FUR	Mph/	
	15:00	2:00	First 10% - FUR	Mph/	
	18:00	3:00	First 50% - FUR	Mph/	
	21:00	3:00	Last 50% - FUR	Mph/	
	25:00	4:00	First 50% - PER	Mph/	
	29:00	4:00	First 50% - PER	Mph/	
	33:00	4:00	Last 50% - PER	Mph/	
	36:00	3:00	Last 50% - PER	Mph/	
	39:00	3:00	PER - FUR	Mph/	
	42:00	3:00	Last 50% - FUR	Mph/	
	45:00	3:00	First 50% - FUR	Mph/	
	50:00	5:00	First 10% - FUR - RHR +	Mph/	

PERSONAL AEROBIC ROUTINES

40-MINUTE CARDIOVASCULAR MOVEMENT
(+10 MINUTE WARM-UP/COOLDOWN= 50 MINUTE TOTAL)

FOR FAT BURNING AND SPORTS/PEAK PERFORMANCE

Name: _____

Age: _____ Gender: _____

ACTIVITY: _____

FUR - Fat-Utilization Rate   PER - Performance Enhancement Rate   SUR - Sugar-Utilization Rate

FUR: _____   PER: _____   SUR: _____

| MOVING ZONE LEVELS | TIME (Per Stage) | HEART RATE | SPEED/INCLINE OR LEVEL/RPM | HEART RATE (Real) |
TIME (Elapsed)				
0:00	0:00	Resting Heart Rate+	0Mph 0	
5:00	5:00	Below - FUR	Mph	
7:00	2:00	Near - FUR	Mph	
9:00	2:00	Nearer - FUR	Mph	
11:00	2:00	First 1% - FUR	Mph	
13:00	2:00	First 50% - FUR	Mph	
15:00	2:00	First 50% - PER	Mph	
17:00	2:00	SUR	Mph	
19:00	2:00	PER - FUR	Mph	
21:00	2:00	PER	Mph	
24:00	3:00	SUR	Mph	
26:00	2:00	PER - FUR	Mph	
28:00	2:00	PER	Mph	
32:00	4:00	SUR	Mph	
34:00	2:00	PER - FUR	Mph	
36:00	2:00	PER	Mph	
41:00	5:00	SUR	Mph	
45:00	4:00	PER - FUR	Mph	
50:00	5:00	FUR - RHR+	Mph	

13 | FOR HEALTHY MUSCLES, YOU MUST RESIST

The Law of Adaptation and Resistance Exercise

Due to the Law of Adaptation, muscles that are continuously under "resistance" become stronger, leaner, and better developed. Muscles adapt to whatever force you apply to them. Or don't. If you consistently put a strain on a certain muscle group, it will adapt by getting more physically powerful, more tone, and it will change its shape. If you consistently do not put strain on your muscles, they become weaker, flabbier, and shapeless.

Again, to be healthy, lean muscle mass must increase, and fat must decrease. While aerobic exercise will cause some resistance to the set of muscles being used, it is not enough. Resistance needs to be applied throughout the entire body so you remove fat and increase leanness in all or most of the muscles.

Resistance exercise occurs when you apply sustained or repetitive strain (resistance) to muscle. The most effective way to create resistance against the muscles and thus produce predictable results is a properly applied weight-lifting program.

ANAEROBICS

Anaerobics, or exercise "without air," are activities like weight lifting, sprinting, or any exercise done hard and for under fifteen minutes. Anaerobic exercises typically are not going to aid the BBG cardiovascular system or cause a great deal of fat burning. However, anaerobic exercises still have benefits to the cardiovascular system and body fat levels due to the effect of creating more quality muscle tissue out of what used to be poor-quality fat tissue.

BBG Owner's Caution: Use It or Lose It

Unfortunately, the BBG is not very forgiving when it comes to the Law of Adaptation to resistance exercise. Within as little as forty-eight hours after performing resistance exercise, the muscles involved begin to atrophy. When muscles atrophy, that means they get smaller, weaker, or, in other words, go away. God has set it up so that it is important that you consistently apply some sort of resistance to your muscles.

Remember the law of *"use it, or lose it."* No resistance, no muscles.

YOU NEED TO MOVE, NO "BONES" ABOUT IT!

Through the Law of Adaptation (the law of "use it or lose it"), the bones, like muscle, gain strength or gain weakness depending on how much pressure is applied. When you move, you place pressure on the bones and they adapt by building up more bone tissue. The more pressure, the more bone.

For instance, martial artists will actually spend time tapping their fists against a brick or other hard surface to build up extra bone in their hands and wrists so they can deliver a more intense blow.

Eating foods that contain more calcium, magnesium, and other minerals is important for building bone; however, it is *movement* that actually causes these elements to be laid down on the bone.

While there is some natural tendency for the BBG to lose bone as it gets older, the most significant reason for diminished bone mass is the natural tendency of people to also stop moving as they get older. If you keep moving, bone keeps growing.

When women lack regular movement, this loss of bone is so severe it can be not only unhealthy, it can be deadly. Due to the hormonal changes women go through as they age, without exercise the bones can become so weak and brittle that it can lead to fractures and even death.

You need to keep moving, *no bones about it.*

BBG Owner's Tip for Exercising for Life

The Owner's Manual 3-Minute Body Parts routines that follow will show you how to achieve muscle strength, tone, leanness, and more healthy bones in workouts that are as little as ten minutes long. These short but extremely effective workouts fit into any lifestyle or fitness level. This makes it possible to exercise not just today, or for the next ninety days, but for *life.*

THE LANGUAGE OF RESISTANCE MOVEMENT THROUGH WEIGHT TRAINING

The world of resistance weight training brings with it its own unique and special vocabulary. Such terms need to be defined before a proper understanding of the weight resistance program can occur. They include the following:

Repetitions (or Reps)

In the vernacular of weight training, a repetition is defined as how many times you *do* the specified exercise. If you lift a weight 12 times, that is 12 repetitions, or "reps."

Sets

A set is how many separate times you perform the repetitions of the exercise. For instance, 3 "sets" of 12 repetitions is performing 12 repetitions, 3 separate times.

Failure

Doing an exercise until "failure" means performing a "set" until you literally cannot perform even one more "rep."

Intensity

Intensity means an exercise is more challenging. However, be forewarned, that doesn't mean you have to use heavy weights or perform workouts that are unsafe or more painful.

While adding heavier weights to your sets will increase intensity, too much weight can also cause pain and injury. The safest way to increase the intensity of a workout is to shorten the time between "sets" or shorten the time between each exercise. In this way, intensity not only makes your workouts more effective, it makes them more time efficient as well.

The more intense your workouts are, the faster you will see results!

Posture + Stretching + Counting + Breathing = *Safe and Effective Exercise!*

HOW TO STAND: PERFECT POSTURE = PERFECT TECHNIQUE

All exercise and stretching, as well as all movement in life, needs to be performed as close to *perfect posture* as possible. God designed the body using all of the vast, highly technical laws of science, mathematics, and physics in order for your BBG to best deal with gravity. When maintaining your posture, the muscles, joints, and bones are at their strongest and most stable. This will allow them to be able to withstand large or repetitive forces without suffering injury.

Perfect Posture

- (A) The head is up and back so the ears line up over the shoulders, and the arc (lordosis or "C" curve) in the neck is maintained.
- (B) Shoulders are rolled back in the joints.
- (C) Upper back is flat and not arched or humped.
- (D) Belly button is out and hips back so you have an arc (lordosis/"C" curve like the neck) in your lower back, called the "weight lifter's arch."
- (E) Knees are slightly bent to provide shock absorption.

Remember to maintain this posture during *all* stretches and exercises. Any exercise or stretch that calls for a disruption of posture means it is unhealthy or you are doing it wrong.

HOW TO STRETCH

Due to sitting, driving, working on the computer, getting out of shape, and the effects of gravity, certain muscles get too short or too tight. This can create an injury during lifting or cause you to develop joint pain and degeneration over time.

In order to compensate for the natural muscle shortening that occurs due to our modern, unnatural lifestyles, stretching is critical to perform before, during, and after every workout.

BBG Owner's EBG Reminder
Always stretch before and after each cardiovascular or resistance workout.

Short Muscles and Their Stretches

Hamstrings: While standing, put your foot up on a chair or bench. Keeping perfect posture (head up/shoulders back/weight lifter's arc in your back), bend down slightly toward your foot, making sure to keep your head and shoulders up. You should feel a stretch in the back of your leg and calf.

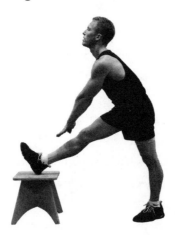

Calves: Stand two to three feet away from a wall and lean against it while keeping your back and legs straight so you are bending forward at the ankle only. You should feel a stretch at the Achilles tendon and calf muscles.

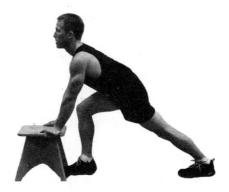

Chest Muscles/Front Shoulders: Stand by a wall or in a doorway and put your hand against it at eye level. Move or lean forward away from your hand until your arm is straight and being pulled back enough to cause a stretch in the chest and shoulder muscles. Change the level of your hand to below the waist and above your head in order to perform this stretch at three different angles.

Front of Neck: Roll your shoulders back, pull your chin in, and then roll your head back so you are looking up at the ceiling behind you. This is done to stretch the front of the neck. The muscles and ligaments in the front of the neck get tight due to the forward head posture created by driving, watching TV, or sitting at a desk or computer.

Hold all stretches for ten to fifteen seconds, back off slightly, take a deep breath in, and then let it out while you repeat the stretch for another ten to fifteen seconds. Each

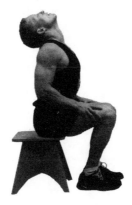

time you go back down while breathing out, you should be able to stretch farther. Do each stretch at least three separate times to achieve the maximum benefit.

HOW TO BREATHE WHILE LIFTING

Breathe in on the eccentric contraction (while you are lowering or releasing the weight) and breathe out on the concentric contraction (while you are lifting the weight).

HOW TO COUNT WHILE LIFTING

Count "1, 2," on the concentric contraction (when lifting). Count "1, 2, 3, 4," on the eccentric contraction (when releasing or lowering the weight).

14 | RESISTANCE EXERCISES

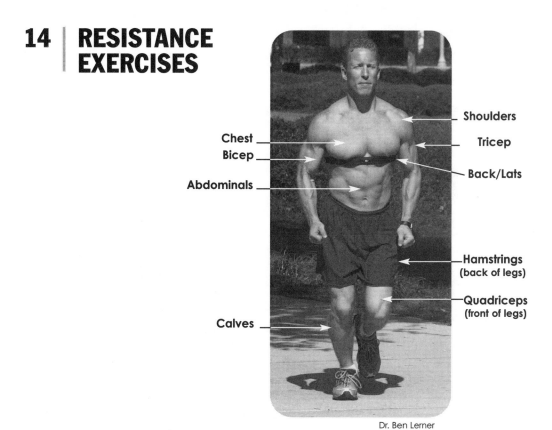

Dr. Ben Lerner

THE LOWER BODY

Lower-body resistance movements should address six main areas for women, and four main areas for men. They are as follows: **Quadriceps** (the muscles on the front of the upper leg); **Hamstrings** (the muscles on the back of the upper leg); **Calves** (the muscles on the back of the lower leg); and **Gluteus muscles** (the muscles you sit on).

Women typically have to include additional movements for **Inner Thigh Muscles** (the inside of the upper leg) and **Outer Thigh Muscles** (the outside of the upper leg). These are areas where they tend to store fat, while men typically do not.

Lower-Body Exercises

("*" Denotes Preferred Exercise by God)

Squats and Lunges

Squats and lunges are the most effective way to build lean muscle and strength in the body's largest and most significant areas: quadriceps, gluteus, hamstrings, and inner/outer thighs.

*One-Legged Squat (Quadriceps, Hamstrings, Glutes)

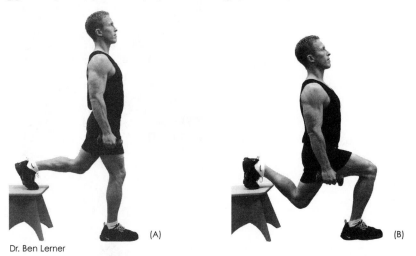

(A) (B)

Dr. Ben Lerner

I like the one-legged squat because it is a natural movement and creates very little pressure in the shoulders and lower back. This exercise takes the hips and knees through a more natural range of motion.

(A) Position: To perform a one-legged squat, find a surface (bench or chair) that is approximately knee height. Stand, in posture, in front of the surface and place one foot on top of it, keeping the bench or chair behind you.

(B) Movement: Squat down with your other leg until the back of it is parallel to the floor and at an approximate 90 degree angle to your lower leg and calf. Then stand back up to the starting position.

Breathe in, "1, 2, 3, 4," on the way down, and breathe out, "1, 2," on the way up.

Tip: To elevate the difficulty or intensity level, you can perform this exercise while holding weights in your hands and increasing the weight as you get stronger.

Standard Squat

This exercise is a more unnatural type of movement that puts a tremendous amount of pressure on the shoulders, lower back, and knees. If you are having trouble with any of these areas, avoid the two-legged squat. It is the easiest exercise during which to sustain an injury if done incorrectly.

Position: Stand with your feet slightly more than shoulder width apart, in posture, holding a barbell just behind your shoulders.

Movement: Maintaining perfect posture and looking up, squat down as if getting ready to sit until the back of your legs are parallel to the floor and at a 90-degree angle to your calves. Your lower legs and calves must remain close to perpendicular to the floor, with your knees remaining directly above your ankle and not out in front of your toes. Then stand back up to the starting position.

Breathe in, "1, 2, 3, 4," on the way down, and breathe out, "1, 2," on the way up.

Caution: When performing a one- or two-legged squat, do not let your knee or knees get out in front of your toes or bend over and lose perfect posture. If you feel any pain or pulling sensation in your back, knees, or hips, stop the exercise immediately and consult a health professional.

*Lunges (Quadriceps, Hamstrings, Glutes)

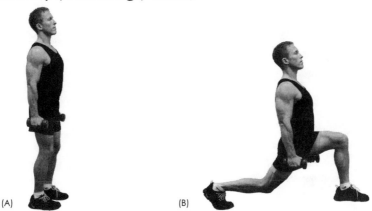

(A) (B)

A lunge is another excellent, safe, and natural movement for working the legs, glutes, hips, and thighs.

(A) Position: Stand in good posture with or without weights in your hands, depending on strength and experience.

(B) Movement: Take a long step forward, bringing your center line (your groin) toward the back of your front ankle and bending your front knee until that upper leg is at a 90-degree angle to your lower leg. The front lower leg must remain close to perpendicular to the floor, with your knee over your foot and ankle but not out over your toes. Your back knee should bend down until it is two to three inches above the floor and your back toes are bent. Hold that position for a moment. Then push back with your front foot so you are back to the starting position. Repeat 10–15 times with that leg and then switch legs.

Breathe in, "1, 2, 3, 4," on the way down, and breathe out, "1, 2," on the way up.

Tip: To make the move more challenging, after completing the lunge, instead of pushing with your front foot back into a standing position, bring your back foot forward as if you were walking. Then step out again, always bringing your back foot up so you end up walking across the floor.

Additional Tip: A lunge is slightly easier on the knees than a one-legged squat, so it is a good exercise for those with knee issues.

Caution: Do not allow your back knee to hit the ground or your front knee to extend over your toes.

Leg Extension (Quadriceps)

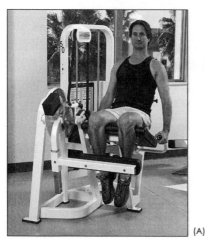
(A)

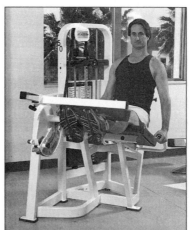
(B)

Dave Phillips

This exercise is not considered an EBG because it isolates one muscle group rather than being a natural movement that recruits several. However, leg extensions are great exercises because they strengthen the muscles surrounding the knee that typically become weak due to the modern lifestyle disease of sitting too much.

(A) Position: Sit on a leg extension machine and slide your legs under the roller pads. Hook your ankles underneath the pads so the pads are resting on top of your lower shin area. Grab the handles or the sides of the bench.

(B) Movement: With your toes pointed out, lift your legs until your knees are straight. Hold this for a second while squeezing your quadriceps (thigh muscles), then lower the weight slowly back to the starting position.

Breathe out, "1, 2," on the way up, and breathe in, "1, 2, 3, 4," on the way down.

Tip: If you do not have access to a leg extension machine, you can do this at home using a paint can filled with sand. Sit in a chair and hook your foot under the handle and perform the exercise one leg at a time.

Caution: Sit in good posture, and do not lift your bottom off the seat.

Leg Curl (Hamstrings)

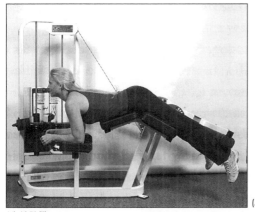

(A)　　　　　　(B)

Vicki Phillips

(A) Position: Lie facedown on a leg curl machine and put your ankles under the roller pad so it is resting on the backs of your lower ankles. Keep your head arched up slightly and grab the handles or the sides of the bench you are lying on.

(B) Movement: Bend your legs until the roller pad hits the top of your hamstrings (the backs of your legs). Hold that position for a second while squeezing your hamstrings, and then slowly lower the weight back down to the starting position.

Breathe out, "1, 2," on the way up, and breathe in, "1, 2, 3, 4," on the way down.

Dumbbell Hamstring Curl

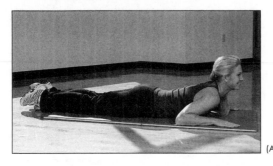
(A)

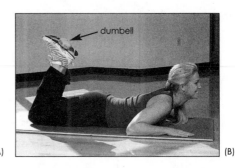
dumbell

(B)

Tip: If you do not have access to a hamstring curl machine, this can be done lying facedown on the floor while holding a dumbbell between your feet, and performing the exercise the same way. It can also be done on a bench with a partner placing and removing dumbells from between your feet.

Caution: Do not allow your hips to rise up off the bench or floor.

Dumbbell Straight-Leg Dead Lifts (Hamstrings and Lower Back)

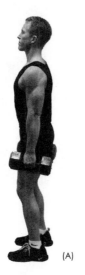
(A)

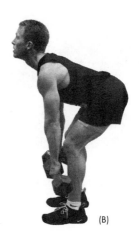
(B)

(A) Position: Stand, holding one dumbbell in each hand, with your knees a little more than slightly bent, your palms facing your legs, and an intense focus on posture (particularly your "weight lifter's arch").

(B) Movement: Maintaining correct posture in your lower back, shoulders, and neck, lower the weights toward the floor. Stop before the weights touch the ground and/or before you feel that you must begin to lose your weight lifter's arch, arch or hump your upper back, or drop your head and shoulders forward. Once you get to this point, reverse the movement, standing back up to the starting position. During this movement, you should feel a good stretch in your hamstrings, particularly where they tie into your gluteus muscles.

Breathe in, "1, 2 ,3, 4," on the way down, and breathe out, "1, 2," on the way up.

Tip: This exercise can be done with a barbell. However, the barbell makes it more difficult to maintain good posture and protect your lower back.

Caution: This exercise is safe for the lower back only when done properly. Make sure to maintain good posture throughout this exercise. Keep the "weight lifter's arch" in your lower back, do not arch or hump your upper back, and do not drop your head forward.

Abduction (Outer Thigh)

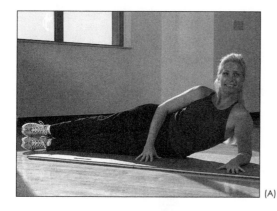
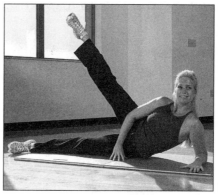

(A)

(B)

(A) Position: Lie on your side, with your knees slightly bent and your legs lying on top of each other.

(B) Movement: Lift your top leg straight up toward the ceiling as high as you can, using your outer thigh and hip muscles. Hold the position for one second, and then slowly lower back down to the starting position.

Breathe out, "1, 2," on the way up, and breathe in, "1, 2, 3, 4," on the way down.

Adduction (Inner Thigh)

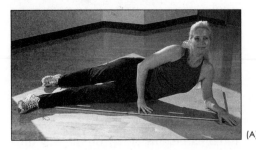 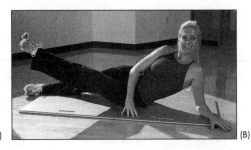

(A) (B)

(A) Position: Lie on your side, with your bottom leg placed straight out in front of your upper leg.

(B) Movement: Lift the bottom leg, using your inner thigh and hip muscles. Hold the position for one second, then lower slowly.

Breathe out, "1, 2," on the way up, and breathe in, "1, 2, 3, 4," on the way down.

Tip: To make abduction and adduction more challenging, wear an ankle weight.

Additional Tip: Abduction/adduction can also be performed on a machine.

*One-Legged Calf Raise (Calves)

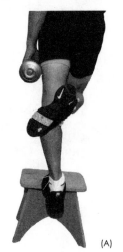 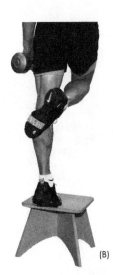

(A) (B)

(A) Position: Start by standing with the ball of your right foot on a surface that is several inches off the ground. Hold a dumbbell (or no weight for beginners) in your right hand, and hold on to something else with your left hand to give you balance.

(B) Movement: Lower your right heel slowly toward the ground as far as possible and then lift up toward the ceiling as far as possible. When you get to the top of the movement, squeeze your calf muscle for one second, and then slowly lower your heel back to the bottom.

Breathe out, "1, 2," on the way up, and breathe in, "1, 2, 3, 4," on the way down.

Seated Calf Raise (Calves)

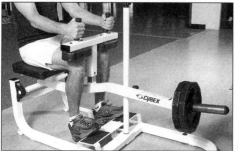 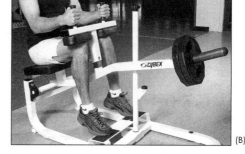

(A) (B)

Position: Sit down in perfect posture on a seated calf-raise machine so the balls of your feet are on the foot platform and your knees are underneath the pads.

Movement: Slowly lower your heels as far as you can and then lift the weight up as high as possible. Hold the weight at the top and squeeze your calf muscles for one second. Then slowly lower your heels all the way back to the bottom again.

Breathe out, "1, 2," on the way up, and breathe in, "1, 2, 3, 4," on the way down.

Tip: A seated calf raise does not work the entire calf muscle. A standing calf-raise machine or one-legged calf raise can be used to better reach the whole calf muscle.

Additional Tip: If you do not have access to a calf machine, you can achieve a similar effect by standing on a book or on a step and lifting yourself up and down using your calf muscles.

Caution: Do not allow your ankles or knees to roll out as you lift up during any calf movement.

THE UPPER BODY

The Muscles Used During an Upper Body Workout

Upper-body resistance movements need to concentrate on the following six areas:

Chest, Triceps (the muscles on the backside of the upper arm), **Biceps** (the muscles on the front side of the upper arm), **Shoulders** (deltoids and rear deltoids), **Back** (lats), and **Abdominals.**

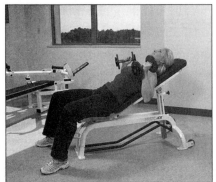

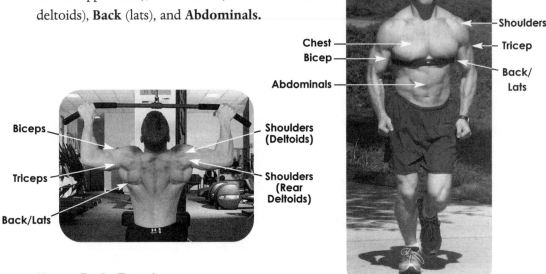

Upper-Body Exercises

("*" Denotes Preferred Exercise by God)

Bench presses are a good way to hit several muscle groups all at one time. They work the chest, shoulders, and triceps all at once. I prefer dumbbells because they allow more natural freedom of movement than barbells do. This makes them safer, more effective, and great EBG. On the following pages, you will find several other helpful Exercises by God:

Incline Dumbbell Flye Press (Chest, Shoulders, Triceps)

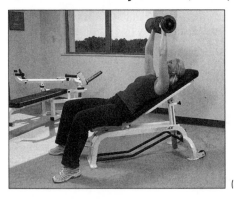

(A)

(B)

(A) Position: Holding two dumbbells, lie back on a bench that is at a slight incline (approximately 20–40 degrees). Hold the weights so your palms are facing toward you and your elbows are bent so your hands are just above your body.

(B) Movement: Push the weights straight up over the sternum/chin area while rotating your hands so your palms begin to face away from you and your thumbs are facing each other. Push the weights all the way up until just before your elbows are locked. Touch the weights together slightly and hold that position for one second. Then slowly lower the weight while rotating your hands so your palms are again facing you and you are back in the starting position.

Breathe out, "1, 2," on the way up, and breathe in, "1, 2, 3, 4," on the way down.

Flat Dumbbell Flye Press (Chest, Shoulders, Triceps)

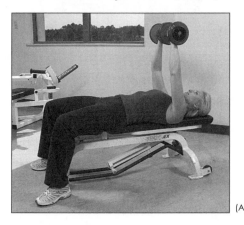
(A)

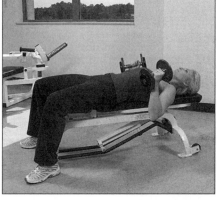
(B)

(A) Position: Holding two dumbbells, lie back on a flat bench. Like the incline flye press, hold the weights so your palms are facing toward you and your elbows are bent so your hands are just above your body.

(B) Movement: Push the weights straight up over the sternum/chin area while rotating your hands so your palms begin to face away from you and your thumbs are facing each other. Push the weights all the way up until just before your elbows are locked. Touch the weights together and hold that position for a second. Then slowly lower the weight while rotating your hands so your palms are again facing you and you are back in the starting position.

Breathe out, "1, 2," on the way up, and breathe in, "1, 2, 3, 4," on the way down.

Tip: By internally rotating the hands on the way up (bringing your thumbs toward each other), you get more use out of the chest muscles.

Caution: Do not lift your head or hips off the bench while you are lifting.

Incline Flyes (Chest)

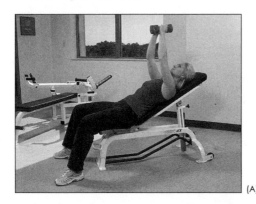

(A)

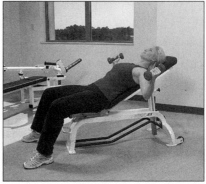

(B)

(A) Position: Hold a dumbbell in each hand and lie down on a bench that is placed at a slight incline. Hold the dumbbells up over your body with your palms facing each other and your elbows slightly bent.

(B) Movement: Slowly lower the weight down and out in an arclike movement so the weights are coming down away from your body. Lower your elbows until they are even with the bench. Hold for a count of two and then return to the top, maintaining the same arclike path you made on the way down. At the top of the movement, squeeze your chest muscles together for a count of two before again lowering the weight.

Breathe out, "1, 2," on the way up, and breathe in, "1, 2, 3, 4," on the way down.

Caution: Do not let your elbows drop down below the bench or allow your arms to go out straight at the bottom of the movement.

*Incline or Flat Push-Up (Chest, Shoulders, Triceps)

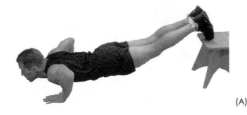

(A)

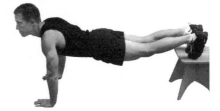

(B)

(A & B) Movement: With your feet on the floor or up on a raised surface, perform push-ups, keeping your head up and your back straight.

Breathe out, "1, 2," on the way up, and breathe in, "1, 2, 3, 4," on the way down.

Tip: To make this movement easier, you can do the push-ups from your knees.

Additional Tip/Caution: Do not let your hips sag down below your body or lift up above your body.

*Barbell Curl (Biceps)

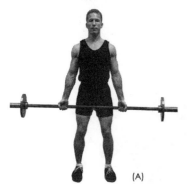 (A)
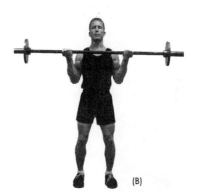 (B)

(A) Position: Stand in correct posture, holding a barbell with your hands just slightly more than shoulder width apart.

(B) Movement: Maintain perfect posture, keeping your elbows at your sides, and curl the weight up. At the top of the movement, squeeze your biceps for a count of two, and then slowly lower the weight back to the starting position.

Breathe out, "1, 2," on the way up, and breathe in, "1, 2, 3, 4," on the way down.

*Dumbbell Curl (Biceps)

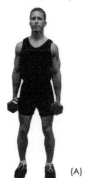 (A)
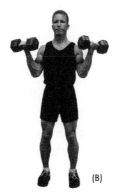 (B)

(A) Position: Stand in posture, holding a dumbbell in each hand with your palms facing toward you.

(B) Movement: Using one arm, curl the weight while rotating your palm and thumb out away from your body. At the top of the movement, squeeze your biceps for a count of two, and then lower the weight while rotating your palm back down into the starting position. Repeat the movement using the other arm.

Breathe out, "1, 2," on the way up, and breathe in, "1, 2, 3, 4," on the way down.

Tip: By rotating your hands, you get more use out of the biceps muscles.

Hammer Curl (Biceps)

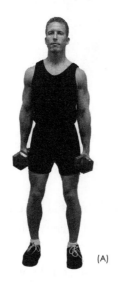 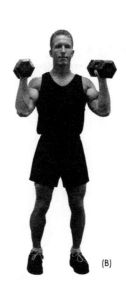

(A)   (B)

(A) Position: Stand in posture, holding a dumbbell in each hand with your palms facing toward you.

(B) Movement: Using one arm at a time, curl the weight up while keeping your palm facing your body. At the top of the movement, squeeze your biceps for a count of two, and then lower the weight back down into the starting position. Repeat the movement using the other arm.

Breathe out, "1, 2" on the way up, and breathe in, "1, 2, 3, 4," on the way down.

Caution: Do not lean far back or use momentum by swaying to lift the weight. Also, do not dig your elbows into your rib cage for leverage.

*Tricep Pushdown—Rope or Bar (Triceps)

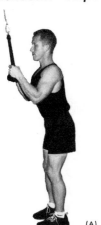
(A)

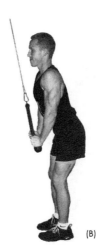
(B)

I like to use a rope if available for this movement in order to get a fuller range of motion out of the triceps. If a rope is not available, a slightly bent bar can be used to get almost the same effect.

(A) Position: Using a cable machine, grab the rope or bar with your palms facing down. The cable must be high enough so your hands are at shoulder level. Keeping the proper straight arch in your back, bend forward very slightly and pull your hands down just below shoulder level, making sure to keep your wrists straight.

(B) Movement: Push the rope or bar down toward your legs, using only your triceps and without moving the rest of your body. Push down until you completely lock out your elbows. If you are using a rope, extend your hands out past your legs. At the bottom of the movement, squeeze your triceps for a count of two before slowly raising the rope or bar back up to the starting position.

Breathe out, "1, 2," on the way down, and breathe in, "1, 2, 3, 4," on the way back up.

Caution: Do not bend over and recruit your shoulders or chest to get the weight down.

One-Arm Standing Triceps Extension (Triceps) *(example on following page)*

(A) Position: Stand, holding one dumbbell straight up over your head with your palm angled slightly in toward your head and your elbow angled slightly out.

(B) Movement: Lower the weight slowly behind your head, keeping your elbow angled slightly out so you do not have to bend your head forward out of posture to get the weight behind it. Lower the weight down as far as you can and then lift it back up

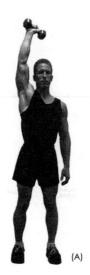

(A)

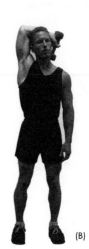

(B)

to the starting position. When you are back up at the top, squeeze your triceps for a count of 2 before performing the movement again.

Breathe out, "1, 2," on the way up, and breathe in, "1, 2, 3, 4," on the way down.

Caution: Do not bend your head down on this or any movement. This can cause neck strain or injury.

*One-Arm Bent Triceps Extension (Triceps)

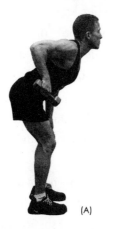

(A)

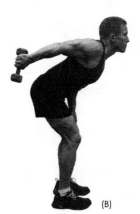

(B)

(A) Position: Stand, holding a dumbbell with your palm facing your body and then bend at the waist, keeping good posture with your back straight and your head up. Place your other hand on your knee or another surface for balance. With the arm holding the dumbbell, lift your elbow straight up and back until your upper arm (bicep/tricep) is parallel to the floor and your elbow is bent at a 90-degree angle.

(B) Movement: Using your triceps, extend the weight back behind you until your elbow is locked out and your entire arm is parallel with the floor. At the top of the lift, squeeze your triceps for a count of 2 before lowering the weight back down to the starting position.

Breathe out, "1, 2," as you extend the weight, and breathe in, "1, 2, 3, 4," as you bring it back down.

Tip: You can also do this by placing your knee on a bench on the same side as the hand holding the weight and placing the other hand down at the end of the bench.

Caution: Do not swing the weight or use momentum from your body to lift it up.

Reverse Bench Dip (Triceps)

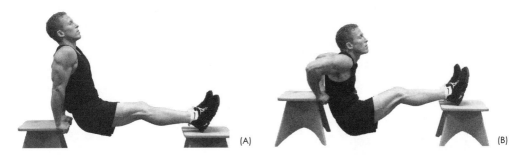

(A) (B)

(A) Position: Place two benches or chairs approximately half a body length apart. Sit on one bench or chair while facing the other. Place your palms on the bench or chair you are sitting on while putting your feet out the other with your knees slightly bent. Then slide your bottom off of the surface you are sitting on and, using your triceps, lift yourself up by locking out your arms.

(B) Movement: Lower your bottom down toward the floor until your upper arm is parallel to the floor. Then straighten your arms back out to return to the beginning position.

Breathe in, "1, 2, 3, 4," on the way down, and breathe out, "1, 2," on the way up.

Tip: You can have someone apply pressure to your shoulders to make the move more challenging.

Caution: Do not lower yourself too far down toward the floor.

Triangle Push-Up (Triceps)

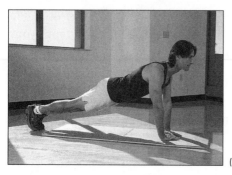 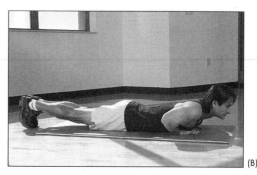

(A)   (B)

(A) Position: Make a triangle out of your hands by putting your thumbs and index fingers together.

(B) Movement: Do push-ups from the floor, with your feet up on a bench, or from your knees, if you are a beginner, by lowering your chest into the center of the triangle that you made with your hands.

Breathe in, "1, 2, 3, 4," on the way down, and breathe out, "1, 2," on the way up.

Dumbbell Shoulder Press (Shoulders, Also Assisted by Triceps)

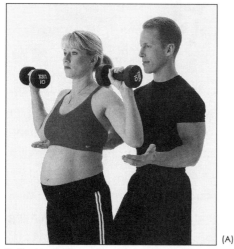 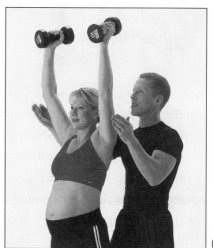

(A)   (B)

Dr. Sheri Lerner (8 months pregnant) with Dr. Ben

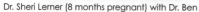

(A) Position: Stand in posture, holding a dumbbell in each hand up at shoulder level with your palms facing inward.

(B) Movement: Press the dumbbells straight up over your head while rotating your palms outward away from you. Lift them up until the dumbbells almost touch, but do not completely lock out your elbows. Then lower the weights back down to the starting position.

Breathe out, "1, 2," on the way up, and breathe in, "1, 2, 3, 4," on the way down.

Lateral Flyes (Shoulders)

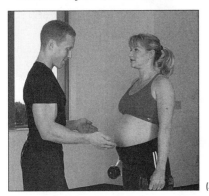 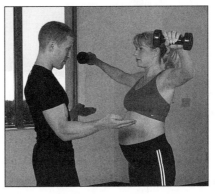

(A) (B)

(A) Position: Stand in posture, holding a dumbbell in each hand down by your legs with your palms facing in towards you.

(B) Movement: Slightly bend your elbows and, using your shoulder muscles, lift your arms out away from your body. Lift up until your hands are at about eye level. Hold the weight there for a count of one and then slowly lower the weight back down to the starting position.

Breathe out, "1, 2," on the way up, and breathe in, "1, 2, 3, 4," on the way down.

Caution: Maintain posture throughout the entire movement, and do not swing or lift the weight using momentum.

*Bent Flyes (Rear Shoulders)**(example on following page)*

(A) Position: Hold a dumbbell in each hand down by your legs with your palms facing in toward your body. Bend forward, keeping your head up, your back in lifting posture, and your knees bent until your chest is just above parallel with the floor.

(B) Movement: Raise the dumbbells up and away from your body by pulling up and out with your elbows until the weights are in line with your shoulders. At the top of the movement, squeeze your shoulder blades together for a count of 2 before slowly lowering them back down to the starting point.

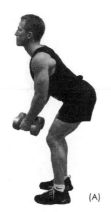
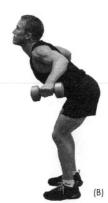

(A)   (B)

Breathe out, "1, 2," as you lift the weight up, and breathe in, "1, 2, 3, 4," as you lower the weight down.

Tip: This is a great movement for overcoming computer posture damage. It builds up the muscles that hold the shoulders back, which will help in overcoming the problems and pain of having stooped shoulders.

Caution: Do not bend over too far or straighten your legs out, or you may strain your lower back. Also, as always, do not use momentum by lifting your body up in order to lift the weight.

Reverse Grip Pulldown (Back)

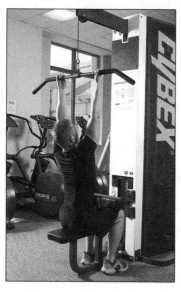
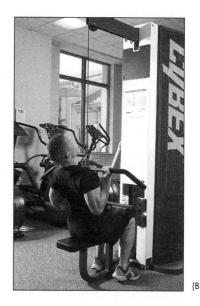

(A)   (B)

(A) Position: Sit in a pull-down machine and reach up under the bar and grip it. Your palms should be facing you, and your arms should be shoulder width apart and stretched up as high as they will go so you are being held down by the knee pads.

(B) Movement: Pull the bar all the way down to your sternum, right below your collarbone, and hold for a count of 2. Do this while squeezing your shoulder blades and shoulders together with your back muscles before going back to the starting position. During the movement, stay in good posture, with your head up and an arch in your lower back.

Breathe out, "1, 2," as you pull the weight down, and breathe in, "1, 2, 3, 4," as you let the weight back up.

Tip: Reverse grips are nice because you can get more range of motion out of your back muscles.

Caution: Do not lean back too far during the movement or use your body to swing the weight down.

*Front-Grip Pulldown (Back)

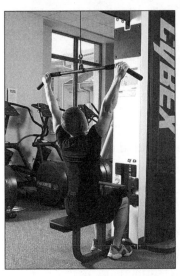 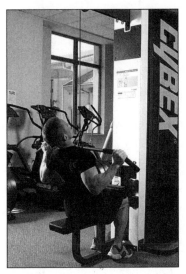

(A)   (B)

(A) Position: Sit in a pull-down machine and reach up over the bar and grip it. Your palms should be facing away from you, and your arms should be 3–6 inches beyond shoulder width apart and stretched up as high as they will go so you are being held down by the knee pads.

(B) Movement: Pull the bar all the way down to your sternum, right below your collarbone, and hold for a count of 2. Do this while squeezing your shoulder blades and shoulders together with your back muscles before going back to the starting position. During the movement stay in good posture, with your head up and an arch in your lower back.

Breathe out, "1, 2," as you pull the weight down, and breathe in, "1, 2, 3, 4," as you let the weight back up.

Caution: A popular way to do pulldowns is to pull the bar behind your neck. This type of pulldown should be avoided as it creates bad posture and can hurt your neck.

One-Arm Dumbbell Row (Back)

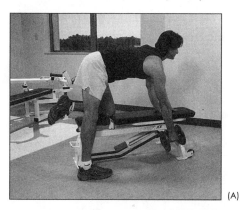 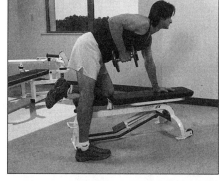

(A) (B)

(A) Position: Holding a dumbbell in one hand, place the opposite hand and the opposite knee on a bench. Bend over so your torso is parallel with the floor, while keeping your head up and the weight lifters arch in your lower back.

(B) Movement: Reach out in front of you with the weight and then, using your back lat muscles, pull your elbow back and up as far as it will go. Hold this lift for a count of 1 at the top, and then slowly lower it until you are reaching out with the weight again. When you are finished, switch hands and leg positions.

Breathe out, "1, 2," as you lift the weight up and out, and breathe in, "1, 2, 3, 4," as you lower the weight down.

Tip: Try to focus on your back by really feeling as if you are rowing.

Caution: Do not use momentum to lift the weight or let your head drop or round your back.

*Pull-Ups/Chin-Ups (Back)

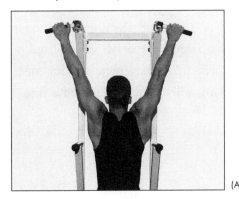 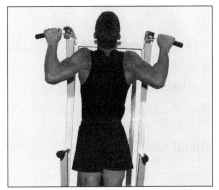

(A) (B)

(A) Position: Hang from a bar with your hands 3–6 inches greater than shoulder width apart and your palms facing away from you in order to do a pull-up, or with your hands shoulder width apart and your palms facing you in order to do a chin-up.

(B) Movement: Simply pull your chin up over the bar, hold for a count of 1, and then lower yourself down all the way.

Breathe out, "1, 2," as you lift yourself up, and breathe in, "1, 2, 3, 4," as you lower yourself back down.

Tip: To help yourself get extra reps, you can put your feet up on a chair or bench or have someone help you up by holding your feet. When you begin to fail, use your legs as leverage.

*Towel Pull-Ups (Back)

This is a pull-up / chin-up for beginners. Put a towel over a door, grab both ends of the towel, and pull yourself up while using your legs for assistance as much as is necessary.

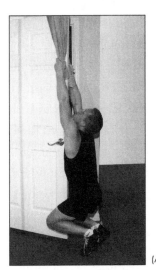 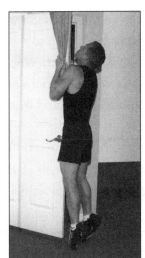

(A) (B)

ABDOMINALS

Your abdomen attaches your sternum to your pelvis. Therefore, the only movements that work your abs are ones that lift the sternum up while the pelvis is stabilized or ones that lift the pelvis up while the sternum is stabilized. Any movement or equipment that does neither, or more than these two movements, will not help your stomach.

When it comes to abs, simplicity is best.

Abdominal Exercises

("★" Denotes Preferred Exercise by God)

Floor Crunch.

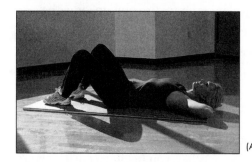 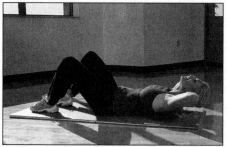

(A)   (B)

(A) Position: Lie flat on your back with your feet flat on the floor. Make a triangle out of your hands and rest your head in the center so your neck is straight and you are looking straight up toward the ceiling.

(B) Movement: Without bending your head or using your arms in any way, lift your head and sternum only a few inches up toward the ceiling using only your stomach muscles. Pretend that an arrow is driving your belly button into the floor while at the same time a string is lifting your nose toward the ceiling. At the top of the movement, "crunch" your abs together for a 2 count and then lower yourself down. *Do not relax your abdominals at the bottom of the move.* When you reach the bottom, hover slightly over the ground and then repeat the movement.

Breathe out, "1, 2," as you lift your sternum. You should be completely out of air as you crunch your abs together for a 2 count. Breathe in, "1, 2, 3, 4," as you lower yourself back toward the floor.

Tip: Hold a weight behind your head as your abdominals get stronger. Remember to still keep your head straight.

Caution: Never hook your legs under anything when doing abdominal routines. You stop using your stomach and start using your back.

*Oblique Crunch

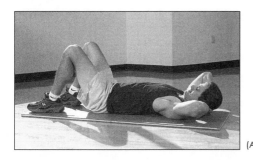
(A)
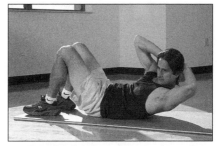
(B)

(A) Position: Lie flat on your back with your feet flat on the floor. Make a triangle out of your hands and rest your head in the center so your neck is straight and you are looking straight up toward the ceiling.

(B) Movement: Lift up toward the ceiling like a regular crunch, but at the top of the movement bring your elbow toward the opposite knee. Repeat for the required number of reps, and then switch to the opposite elbow and knee.

Breathe out, "1, 2," as you lift your sternum and elbow up and across. You should be completely out of air as you crunch your abs together for a 2 count. Breathe in, "1, 2, 3, 4," as you lower yourself back toward the floor.

*Bent-Knee Leg Raise

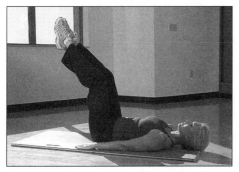
(A)
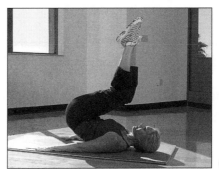
(B)

(A) Position: Lie flat on your back with your hands by your sides, palms down, and your legs bent so your thighs are at a 90-degree angle with your stomach, your knees are bent slightly toward your chest, and your feet are in the air. This can also be done on a bench with hands grabbing the top of the bench.

(B) Movement: Using your abs, lift your pelvis up off the floor toward your nose, then lower back slowly to the starting position.

Breathe out, "1, 2," as you lift your pelvis. Breathe in, "1, 2, 3, 4," as you lower your pelvis back down toward the floor.

Caution: This is not a leg lift. A leg lift uses your lower back. Make sure to keep your legs bent and focus on using your stomach muscles, which are responsible for lifting your pelvis off the ground.

*Side Crunch

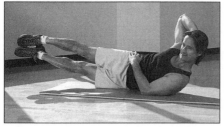 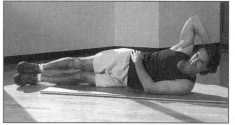

(A)   (B)

(A) Position: Lie on your side with both legs slightly bent and on top of each other, and your top hand reaching down behind your head in order to hold it up.

(B) Movement: Using your side muscles, lift your head and bottom shoulder up off the ground while simultaneously lifting your feet. At the top of the movement, "crunch" your side muscles together for a count of 2 before lowering back down. When you are finished with the required number of reps, roll over and do the other side.

Breathe out, "1, 2," as you lift your head, shoulder, and feet off the floor. You should be completely out of air as you crunch your side abs together for a 2 count. Breathe in, "1, 2, 3, 4," as you lower yourself back toward the floor.

*Side Raise

(A) Position: Lie on your side on top of your elbow, with your top hand palm down on the floor and your bottom hand placed palm down on the floor or on your hip to increase the difficulty.

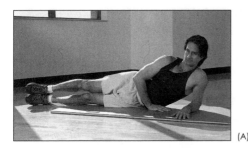
(A)

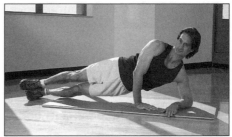
(B)

(B) Movement: Lift your hip up off the ground as far as you can, hold for a count of 2, and then lower.

Breathe out, "1, 2," as you lift your hips off the floor. Breathe in, "1, 2, 3, 4," as you lower your hips back down.

Tip: You can place your top hand on your hip to make the movement more challenging.

GET AN EBG LIFE: RESISTANCE TRAINING AND AEROBIC SCHEDULES

A weekly system of some form of resistance and aerobic Exercise by God is required for good health. Adhering to the following schedules and program outlines will provide the maximum results for whatever level of experience you are at, or for whatever goals you have.

The Best Time of Day to Exercise

- The best time to exercise is anytime. It is always better to do it than not do it.
- The healthiest time to exercise is two to three hours following a meal.
- The time that is most ideal for burning fat and quickly making changes in your body is in the morning, before you have eaten anything, or at least before you have eaten carbohydrates.

Resistance for Maximum Fat-Burning Hypothesis

In the morning, your body is in a fasting state, so it is going to have to use a lot of its stored sugars and fats for energy. When you work out after consuming carbohydrates, your body will burn those sugars for energy instead of using stored sugars and fats.

The Difference Between Men and Women

In the world of weight-resistance movement, there is a unique difference between men and women. Men tend to wear weight in their upper bodies, and women wear it in their lower bodies. Therefore, men need to be more focused on upper-body movements, and women need to be focused on moving their lower bodies.

A basic rule of thumb is this:

• Men should do two upper body workouts for every one lower body workout.
• Women should do two lower body workouts for every one upper body workout.

Women's Schedules

7-Day Women's Basic Health and Body-Shaping Schedule

1 Lower-Body Resistance Routine
1 Upper-Body Resistance Routine
2–3 Aerobic Activities
2 Rest Days

Day 1: Lower Body
Day 2: Aerobic
Day 3: Upper Body
Day 4: Rest
Day 5: Aerobic
Day 6: Rest Or Aerobic
Day 7: Rest
(Repeat)

7-Day Women's Accelerated Health and Body-Shaping Schedule

2 Lower-Body Resistance Routines
1 Upper-Body Resistance Routine
3+ Aerobic Activities
1–2 Rest Days

2 Rest Days
Day 1: Lower Body
Day 2: Aerobic
Day 3: Upper Body
Day 4: Rest
Day 5: Aerobic
Day 6: Lower Body & Aerobic
Day 7: Rest
(Repeat)

1 Rest Day
Day 1: Lower Body
Day 2: Aerobic
Day 3: Upper Body
Day 4: Aerobic
Day 5: Lower Body
Day 6: Aerobic
Day 7: Rest
(Repeat)

BBG Owner's Women's Scheduling Guide

Depending on goals, fitness levels, and amount of inspiration, a woman can do resistance training for her upper body one time a week and lower body as much as two times a week.

When using Quick Sets, muscles need five to six days to recover. Therefore, there should always be five to six days between extremely intense upper- or lower-body workouts.

Women can also choose to do anywhere from two to six days a week of safe, fat-burning zone (FUR) aerobics.

If doing more intense aerobics (PER or SUR), these activities should be limited to three to four days per week to avoid overuse injury.

Men's Schedules

7-Day Men's Basic Health and Body-Shaping Schedule

1 Upper-Body Resistance Routine

1 Lower Body Resistance Routine

2–3 Aerobic Activities

1–2 Rest Days

Day 1: Half Upper Body 1

Day 2: Other Half Upper Body 2

Day 3: Aerobic

Day 4: Lower Body

Day 5: Rest or Aerobic

Day 6: Aerobic

Day 7: Rest

(Repeat)

7-Day Men's Accelerated Health and Body-Shaping Schedule

3 Upper-Body Resistance Routines (Half Each)

1 Lower-Body Resistance Routine

3+ Aerobic Activities

1 Rest Day

Day 1: Half Upper Body 1

Day 2: Half Upper Body 2

Day 3: Aerobic

Day 4: Lower Body

Day 5: Aerobic

Day 6: Half Upper Body 1 and Aerobic

Day 7: Rest

(Repeat, Starting at Half Upper Body 2)

BBG Owner's Men's Scheduling Guide

Depending on goals, fitness levels, or amount of inspiration, a man can do two to four half upper-body resistance training programs and one lower-body resistance training program a week.

If a high-intensity routine, like Quick Sets, is used, the individual muscle groups need five to six days to recover. Therefore, there should always be five to seven days between extremely intense upper- or lower-body workouts.

Men can also choose to do anywhere from two to six days a week of safe, fat-burning-zone (FUR) aerobics a week. If doing more intense aerobics (PER or SUR), these activities should be limited to three to four days per week to avoid overuse injury.

15 | RESISTANCE TRAINING PROGRAMS

3-MINUTE BODY PARTS: THE QUICK-SET PROGRAMS

Starting an exercise program is not nearly as important as *staying* on one. While there are hundreds of movement programs available, it is critical that you begin them with the end in mind. When it comes to exercise you must always ask yourself, "Will I keep it up?" Starting and stopping exercise programs or infrequently exercising does you no good. That is why you must consider everything necessary not just to begin, but to continue.

Body by God: The Owner's Manual for Maximized Living recommends the Quick-Set Programs. These allow you to get a workout in for an individual body part in as little as three minutes. This is the ultimate way to perform resistance training. These routines can be as simple and as short as you need them to be in order to fit them into your schedule or level of motivation on any given day or week. This program can also be performed more or fewer times per week, dependent on how quickly you desire to make changes to the muscles of your BBG. This actually creates the possibility of knowing you will not only exercise consistently this week, or for the next ninety days, but forever.

Due to the type of adaptation the body must make while performing Quick Sets, you are able to create significant changes in the composition (body-fat percentage and muscle tone) of a body part within three minutes. Busy moms, overworked business-men and businesswomen, or students on a tight time schedule can still be extremely effective in their lives and get in shape all at the same time. Using the Quick-Set Programs for three-minute body parts, I and many of my patients, clients, and friends have been able to maintain busy schedules, a high-quality family life, and find plenty of leisure time while still being in the best shape of our lives.

These routines can be used to increase the intensity of your workouts, shorten your workout times, and very safely speed up your results. They are designed so anyone can perform them and make great changes to their BBGs on any level. Whether you are a retired grandma or an aspiring Olympian, there *is* a plan for you on the following pages.

Types of Quick Sets

Decline Set

- Pick one exercise and do it for 8–12 repetitions until failure.
- Rest 5–6 seconds.
- Lower the weight 5–20 pounds and do the exercise again for 6–8 repetitions until failure.
- Rest 5–6 seconds.
- Lower the weight 5–20 pounds again and do another 6–8 repetitions until failure.

Pause Set

- Pick one exercise and do it for 8–12 repetitions until failure.
- Rest 5–6 seconds.
- Using the same weight, do the exercise again until failure.
- Rest 5–6 seconds.
- Repeat this process until you cannot do the exercise for more than 1–2 repetitions.

Monster Set

A Monster Set is when, after performing an exercise for one body part, instead of resting, you immediately perform an exercise for *another* body part. The other body part should be one that was not used while exercising the first body part. For example: chest and biceps, or quadriceps and hamstrings.

Monster Sets are combined with Decline or Pause Sets so you can get a tremendously effective workout done in a very short amount of time. For example, after you perform a Pause Set with the Incline Flye Press for your chest, you can immediately begin performing a Decline Set with Hammer Curls for your biceps.

Cycle Set (1 Cycle = 3–6 Minutes)

To perform a Cycle Set, you set up 3–6 exercises for the same or different body parts. As soon as you are done performing one exercise until failure, you immediately go to the next . . . and then the next. Continue going around the circuit 3 or 4 times.

For example, set up an exercise for quadriceps, an exercise for hamstrings, and an exercise for calves, then do 1 quadriceps exercise then 1 hamstring exercise then 1 calf exercise. Repeat this circuit 3–4 times.

You can also set up 3 exercises for only 1 body part and go around the circuit that way 2–4 times.

Help Reps

Help Reps can be used with any Intensity Set. A Help Rep is performed when a helper or "spotter" stands near you during your set, and when you reach failure they help you to perform 1–2 more repetitions.

MOUNTAIN STRAIGHT SET
(15-20 Minute Workout for Building Muscle Strength, Size, and Power)

It's not 3 minutes, but it *is* a safe way to lift heavier weights and to gain strength.

Up the Mountain *(Beginners perform 1, 2, 3, and 5 only.)*

1. Light to moderate weight with which you can do 12–15 successful repetitions without a hesitation in the movement.
2. Moderate weight with which you can do 10–12 successful repetitions.
3. Moderate to heavy weight with which you can do 8–10 repetitions, struggling with the last 1–2 repetitions.
4. Heavy weight with which you perform 6–8 repetitions struggling, and potentially need assistance with the last 2 repetitions.

5. To increase muscle size or power, you can do 2- to 4- or even 1- to 2-repetition sets (for power and explosion sports).

Down the Mountain

Moderate weight with which you can perform 10 difficult repetitions, possibly needing assistance on the last repetition.

Mountain Straight Sets

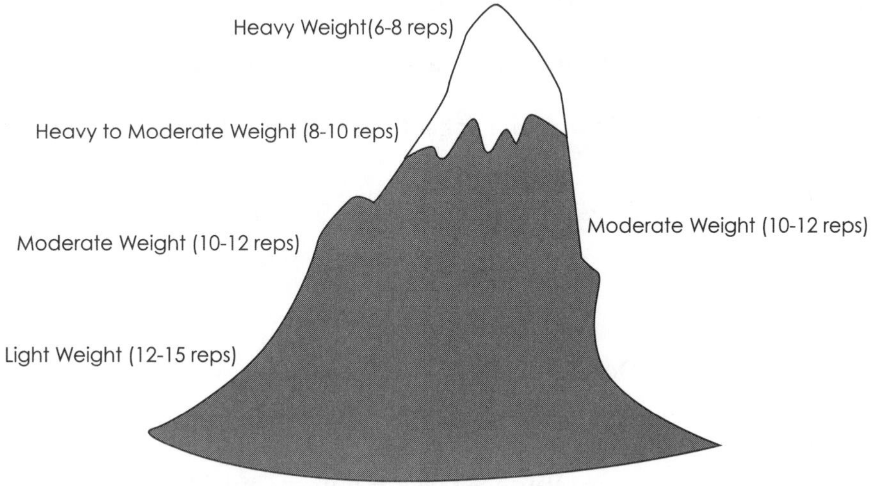

Heavy Weight(6-8 reps)

Heavy to Moderate Weight (8-10 reps)

Moderate Weight (10-12 reps)

Moderate Weight (10-12 reps)

Light Weight (12-15 reps)

3-MINUTE BODY PARTS AND SAMPLE WORKOUTS

Decline and Pause Sets allow you to complete an exercise for a particular body part in approximately 3 minutes. Therefore, a workout consisting of 1 exercise per body part for 3 body parts would take only about 10 minutes, which includes setup time. Workouts become 3 minutes longer or shorter as you do more or less body parts.

Combining Decline and Pause Sets by using the Monster Set drastically decreases your exercise time while drastically increasing the results!

1-Day Sample Upper-Body Workout for Women

3-Minute Body Parts for 6 Parts (20-Minute Workout)

Chest and bicep workout together using the Monster Set Format
- Incline Dumbbell Flye Press: Decline Set with Barbell Curl: Pause Set

Triceps and abdominal workout together using the Monster Set Format
- One-Arm Triceps Extension: Decline Set with Abdominal Crunch: Decline Set Do crunches using a weight behind the head (OR Pause Set if you are unable to use weight)

Back and shoulder workout together using the Monster Set Format
- Front Pulldowns: Decline Set with Lateral Flyes: Decline Set

2-Day Sample Upper-Body Workout for Men

3-Minute Body Parts for 3 Parts (10-, 20-, or 30-Minute Workout)

DAY 1: Half upper-body workout (chest, biceps, and triceps)
10-Minute Workout:
Chest and bicep workout together using the Monster-Set Format.
- Incline Dumbbell Flye Press: Decline Set with Barbell Curl: Pause Set

Triceps
- Triceps Pushdown: Decline Set

For 20-Minute Workout, Add:
- Flat Dumbbell Flye Press: Pause Set *with* Hammer Curl: Decline Set
- One-Arm Triceps Extension: Pause Set

For 30-Minute Workout, Add:
- Push-Ups: Pause Set *with* Dumbbell Curl Pause Set
- Reverse Bench Dips: Pause Set

DAY 2: Half Upper-Body Workout (shoulders, back, and abdominals)
10-Minute Workout:
Back and Shoulder Workout together using the Monster-Set Format
- Reverse Grip Pulldown: Decline Set *with* Dumbbell Press: Pause Set

Abdominals
- Crunch: Decline Set using a weight behind the head (OR Pause Set if you are unable to use weight)

For 20-Minute Workout, Add:
- Dumbbell Row: Pause Set *with* Lateral Flyes: Decline Set
- Bent Leg Raise: Pause Set

For 30-Minute Workout, Add:
- Pull Ups: Pause Set *with* Bent Flyes: Pause Set
- Side Crunch: Pause Set

1-Day Sample Lower-Body Workout for Women and Men

3-Minute Body Parts for 3 Parts (10-, 20-, and 30-Minute Workouts)

10-Minute Workout:
Quadriceps and Hamstring Workout together using the Monster-Set Format
- One-Legged Squat: Decline Set *with* Straight-Leg Dead Lift: Pause Set

Calves
- One-legged Calf Raise: Decline Set

For 20-Minute Workout, Add:
- Lunge: Decline Set *with* Leg Extensions: Pause Set
- Seated Calf Raises: Pause Set

For 30-Minute Workout, Add:
- *[Women Only]* Abduction/Adduction: Decline Set *with* Hamstring Curls: Decline Set or
- Squats: Decline Set *with* Hamstring Curls: Decline Set
- Standing Calf Raise: Decline Set

Or: 10- or 15-Minute Lower-Body Cycle Set
- One-Legged Squat *then* Hamstring Curl *then* One-Legged Calf Raise (go around 3 or 4 times for 10 or 15 minutes)

For 20- or 30-Minute Cycle Set:
- One-Legged Squat *then* Straight-Leg Dead Lift *then* Seated Calf Raise *then* Leg

Extension *then* Hamstring Curl *then* One-Legged Calf Raise (Go around 3 or 4 times for 20 or 30 minutes)

TIPS FOR EXERCISE LONGEVITY

Following these tips will increase your desire to exercise, reduce or eliminate health problems, and help you stick to your program longer—hopefully forever:

1. *Warm up! Warm up! Warm up!* Do 5–10 minutes of stretching and 1–2 warm-up sets of 12–15 reps with very light weight before beginning your exercises. Stretching, warming up the muscles, and adding weight slowly will drastically reduce or eliminate your chance of injury.
2. Beginners, or people attempting to just maintain or develop some strength and muscle tone, can perform only 1 routine a week for lower body and 1 for upper body.
3. Upper-body workouts can be split in half by both men and women to make them shorter and more time-efficient. For example: chest, biceps, and triceps can be exercised separately from back, shoulders, and abdominals.
4. Change your routines around every week or month so you do not get bored and you avoid plateaus due to your body being used to your routine.
5. If you are suffering injuries regularly or feeling excessively sore, physically exhausted, or burned-out, that means you are overtraining. When this happens, take an extra day or days off and/or lower the intensity of the workouts for a week or two. It also means that you need more hydration and more use of foods that reduce/neutralize acids in the body and a more basic environment. (See "Back to Basics" on page 76 in the Food by God part of your Owner's Manual.)
6. Try these combined routines to save even more time or make EBG even easier.

BBG Owner's Guide to Combining Aerobics, and/or Lower- and Upper-Body Resistance Movements

Perform these activities 3–5 times/week for men and women at FUR moving zone for a minimum of 15 minutes with a 5-minute warm-up and cooldown phase.

- Walking with ankle or hip weights while doing shoulder, bicep, and triceps movements (combines all 3)
- Walking with ankle or hip weights while holding hand weights and doing shoulder, bicep, and triceps movements (combines all 3)
- Doing an aerobics class that uses hand weights while stepping, lunging, and/or bending at the knees (combines all 3)
- Doing yard or housework that requires both leg and arm motions (combines all 3, as long as there are at least 15 minutes of straight activity)
- Riding a stationary piece of cardio equipment that has foot and arm pedals (combines all 3)
- Swimming (combines all 3)

START MOVING FROM WHERE YOU ARE

The true measure of people is not determined so much by where they are, but by where they are going. In the beginning and throughout the *Owner's Manual* programs, it will always be important to just *start moving from where you are*. I know how hard it is to change. Setbacks and errors may have accompanied your last efforts to change and created where you are right now, but do not let them determine where you are going. Just begin and keep moving forward. You don't lose if you fail. You lose only if you quit.

We all have something in common: We win some and we lose some. Mostly, when it comes to permanent change, we lose some. What I am praying for, what I wish I could get on the phone with you every day to inspire, what the world needs, and what God is counting on, is that losing doesn't mean the same thing as stopping.

Not stopping is what makes a person who is doing things for God different from everyone else. Everyone fails. If everything is going your way, you are probably going the wrong way. In fact, if you are really trying to make a difference, you'll fail even more often than the average person.

Failing and quitting make you average for a man or woman.

Failing and continuing make you better for God!

Fail, but never give up. Just start moving where you are.

THE BODY BY GOD 40-DAY PLAN FOR MOVEMENT

The *Body by God* 40-Day Plan in the Life by God section at the end of your *Owner's Manual for Maximized Living* will give you recommendations on starting to apply the Laws of Movement.

Like all elements of the 40-Day Plan, all that is required is that you get 40 percent better for God in 40 days and then continue for as long as you desire to keep moving (staying alive). This means that you are not killing yourself at home or in a gym by trying to create miraculous "before and after" pictures in only two weeks. It means you begin . . . and just keep getting better.

On the other hand, the good news is that if you use the Quick-Set Programs for three-minute body parts, along with properly applying your fat-burning Moving Zones, you will see dramatic changes in the health and appearance of your BBG in a very short period of time. This should inspire you to continue exercising and keep improving for God. (See "Overnight Success" plans on p. 349.)

If the LORD delights in a man's way, he makes his steps firm; though he stumble, he will not fall, for the LORD upholds him with his hand. (Ps. 37:23–24)

The Daily BBG Fitness Program

Body Parts: Hamstrings, Quadriceps, Calves, glutes

	Real Date	Real Time	Intended Date	Intended Time by God
	2/24/03	7 (A.M.)/P.M.	2/24/03	6:30 (A.M.)/P.M.

Types of Sets

Legs:	• Decline - **D** 15 - 5 reps 12 - 5 reps	• Pause - **P** 12 - 0 reps 12 - 0 reps	• Mountain - **M** 15 - 5 reps 12 - 5 reps	• Cycle - **C** 15 - 6 reps 12 - 6 reps	• Monster Set - **MO**

Movements		Type of Set					Real		Intended	
Lower-Body Movements		D	P	M	C	MO	Reps	Weight	Reps	Weight
1 Leg Squat		✓				✓	10, 8, 6	10, 5, 0	12, 10, 8	10, 5, 0
w/Straight Leg Dead Lift			✓			✓	10, 8, 4, 2	30	12, 8, 4, 2	30
1 Leg Calf Raise		✓					15, 12, 10	15, 5, 0	15, 12, 10	20, 10, 0
Leg Extension			✓			✓	12, 10, 6, 2		15, 10, 6, 2	
w/ Hamstring Curl		✓				✓	12, 10, 8	50, 40, 30	15, 12, 10	50, 40, 30
Seated Calf Raise		✓					15, 12, 10	50, 40, 30	15, 12, 10	50, 40, 30
Lunge				✓			12, 10, 6, 10	0, 10, 20, 10	12, 10, 6,10	0, 10, 20, 10

10 Minutes   20 Minutes   30 Minutes

The Daily BBG Fitness Program

Body Parts: 1/2 Upper Body -1 : Chest, Triceps, Biceps.

Real Date	Real Time	Intended Date	Intended Time by God
2/24/03	7:45 (A.M.)/P.M.	2/24/03	7:15 (A.M.)/P.M.

Types of Sets

Legs:	•Decline - **D** 15 - 5 reps 12 - 5 reps
Upper Body:	•Pause - **P** 12 - 0 reps 12 - 0 reps

•Mountain - **M** 15 - 5 reps 12 - 5 reps

•Cycle - **C** 15 - 6 reps 12 - 6 reps

•Monster Set - **MO**

Movements	Type of Set					Real		Intended	
Upper-Body Movements	D	P	M	C	MO	Reps	Weight	Reps	Weight
Incline Dumbell Flye Press	✓				✓	10, 6, 5	45, 35, 30	10, 8, 6	45, 35, 30
w/ Barbell Curl	✓				✓	12, 8, 6	65, 55, 45	12, 8, 6	65, 55, 45
Tricep Pushdown	✓					12, 10, 6	50, 40, 30	12, 10, 8	50, 40, 30
Flat Dumbell Flye Press		✓			✓	8, 6, 4, 2	40	8, 6, 4, 2	40
w/ Hammer Curl		✓			✓	10, 6, 4, 2	30	10, 6, 4, 2	30
Bent Tricep Extension		✓				12, 8, 4, 1	15	12, 8, 4, 2	15
Incline Push-up		✓			✓	20, 12, 6, 2	-	20, 15, 10, 5	-
w/ Bicep Dumbell Curl		✓			✓	10, 5, 2, 1	25	10, 6, 4, 2	25
Reverse Dips		✓				12, 6, 3, 1	-	12, 6, 3, 2	-

10 Minutes

20 Minutes

30 Minutes

The Daily BBG Fitness Program

Body Parts: 1/2 Upper Body - 2 : Shoulders, Back, Abdominals

Real Date	Real Time	Intended Date	Intended Time by God
2/24/03	8:30 (A.M.)/P.M.	2/24/03	8:00 (A.M.)/P.M.

Types of Sets

Legs:
- Decline - **D** 15 - 5 reps
- Mountain - **M** 15 - 5 reps
- Cycle - **C** 15 - 6 reps
- Monster Set - **MO**

Upper Body:
- Pause - **P** 12 - 0 reps
- 12 - 5 reps
- 12 - 6 reps

Movements	Type of Set						Real		Intended	
Upper-Body Movements	**D**	**P**	**M**	**C**	**MO**	**Reps**	**Weight**	**Reps**	**Weight**	
Reverse Grip Pulldown	✓				✓	12, 10, 6	90, 80, 70	12,10, 8	90, 80, 70	
w/ Military Press	✓				✓	12, 10, 8	40, 30, 20	12, 10, 8	40, 30, 20	
Crunch		✓				15, 10, 8, 5	–	15, 10, 8, 6	–	
(10 Minutes)										
Dumbell Row		✓			✓	10, 8, 6, 4	40	12, 10, 8, 6	40	
w/ Lateral Flye		✓			✓	12,10, 8, 4, 2	20	10, 8, 4, 2	20	
Bent Leg Raise		✓				12, 8, 4, 2	–	12,10, 8, 4, 2	–	
(20 Minutes)										
Pullups		✓			✓	8, 4, 2, 1	–	10, 8, 4, 2,1	–	
w/ Bent Shoulder Flye		✓			✓	10, 8, 6, 2	20	10, 8, 6, 2	20	
Oblique Crunch		✓				20,15,10,5, 2	–	20,15,10, 5, 2	–	
(30 Minutes)										

The Daily BBG Fitness Program

Body Parts: _____

Real Date	Real Time	Intended Date	Intended Time by God
_____	_____ A.M./P.M.	_____	_____ A.M./P.M.

Types of Sets
Legs:
Upper Body:

- Decline - **D**
  15 - 5 reps
  12 - 5 reps
- Pause - **P**
  12 - 0 reps
  12 - 0 reps
- Mountain - **M**
  15 - 5 reps
  12 - 5 reps
- Cycle - **C**
  15 - 6 reps
  12 - 6 reps
- Monster Set - **MO**

Movements

Lower Body Movements	Type of Set					Real		Intended	
	D	P	M	C	MO	Reps	Weight	Reps	Weight

10 Minutes 20 Minutes 30 Minutes

The Daily BBG Fitness Program

Body Parts: ....

Real Date	Real Time	Intended Date	Intended Time by God
	.... A.M./P.M.	....	.... A.M./P.M.

Types of Sets

Legs:
Upper Body:

- Decline - **D**
  15 - 5 reps
  12 - 5 reps

- Pause - **P**
  12 - 0 reps
  12 - 0 reps

- Mountain - **M**
  15 - 5 reps
  12 - 5 reps

- Cycle - **C**
  15 - 6 reps
  12 - 6 reps

- Monster Set - **MO**

Movements	Type of Set					Real		Intended	
Upper-Body Movements	D	P	M	C	MO	Reps	Weight	Reps	Weight

10 Minutes

20 Minutes

30 Minutes

PART FOUR | # STRESS MANAGEMENT FOR YOUR BODY BY GOD

16 | PEACE BY GOD

YOUR LIFE IS ON FIRE—WAKE UP AND SMELL THE SMOKE!

To really change your stress levels requires a moment of awakening. It takes a time when you look around you and finally realize that you are not a victim of your crises; you are at the root of them. The challenge is that it is human nature to need to come near to complete and total destruction before we finally stop looking at everyone and everything around us for the answer to our problems and finally start looking at the person looking back at us in the mirror.

If you are like I am, you need lightning to strike twice, make the walls come tumbling down, set your whole world on fire, and fill your entire life with smoke before you ever wake up and say to God, *"Are you talking to me?"*

My most common crises always used to be in the area of relationships. Of course, I always thought the cause of my problems were all these crazy, needy, incompetent people around me. Little did I realize that it was me who was making them crazy, needy, and incompetent. It took pain after pain, broken heart after broken heart, and regret after regret before I ever finally woke up to the fact that the reason I had so much stress from relationships was that I did not know how to relate.

I grew up with parents who loved me. However, they were from the Bronx of New

York, and love in my house was more tough and implied than shown and expressed. As a result, I related to everyone else the same way—by using tough, implied love. Unfortunately, no one seemed to understand this kind of love. I never opened up to anyone, so everyone around me was nervous, insecure, and in need of my attention.

When I finally woke up and smelled the smoke rising off the blazing infernos that were my relationships and clouding every room of my life, I realized I was not the victim of bad relationships, I was the cause of bad relationships. I soon began to take responsibility for my problems. I began to *try* to focus on the needs of others, started staying present and aware of the emotions of the people around me, and worked on expressing love more gently and openly. In time, I was living in a whole new world.

Before I take you through the process of understanding the damaging effects of stress and learning how to overcome it, it is vitally important that you take responsibility for your life. Like me and my relationship problems, you can begin living in a whole new world when you wake up and realize the smoke that is surrounding you is coming from fires that you helped to start.

Stress Management by God will help to pull the matches out of your hand and save you from the slow and painful death of smoke inhalation.

WAKE UP AND SMELL THE DIAPER

When my newborn son came home he brought me incredible joy—with one minor exception: diapers. I do not really know what this is like for most parents, but for me, the diaper years were very painful. My last prepotty-trained memory is of my son filling up the back of his diaper at a local mall. The emotional trauma began for me when, after a thirty-minute search, all I could find was a very small, very dirty bathroom that did not contain a changing station. By the time I opened up his diaper, its contents had been there so long that it had become like tile grout and was serving the same purpose. To make matters worse, when I looked inside the diaper bag it revealed only one diaper and no wet wipes to use as a cleaning apparatus.

Looking to adapt to the situation, I sought out a paper towel or piece of toilet paper, but there was none to be found. At this point, my son was screaming full-blast. I was so frustrated I would have paid a thousand dollars for even one moist towelette. Finally, in desperation, I came up with the ingenious idea of taking out some of the cotton-like stuffing from the diaper and using it as a cleaning tool. Alas, the diaper stuffing didn't work. When I tried to clean him with it, the cotton broke apart into tiny particles. He now looked like he had been tarred and feathered. Needless to say, I was ready for him to be potty trained. The stress came from the fact that he wasn't ready to be potty trained.

When we first started trying to teach my son to use the big-boy bathroom, he did not want to change. After all, the old system was all he had ever known—it was comfortable and seemed to be working out just fine. Things seemed easy. When he had to go, he just went. No need to waste time going into a separate room, taking off his clothes, or even going into the house, for that matter. If he was eating breakfast or out playing with his friends and the need hit, he went. Then suddenly, out of the blue, after using a system that appeared to be working just fine, we suddenly gave him this whole new way of doing things.

We started teaching him that when Mommy and Daddy go in that little room, we actually take off the diaper and go in the bowl of water (to which his first thought was probably that he should stop playing in that thing from now on). We tried to give him information about big boys and girls who don't go in their pants, and that going in your pants was wrong.

To encourage him to accept this new way of life, some days we'd have three or four people standing around him in the bathroom, cheering him on. We'd be screaming, "You can do it!" or "Go, go, go, go! Woohoo!" or "Great job!" Unfortunately, at first, no matter how hard we tried, he would not "wake up and smell the diaper." Therefore, he just kept going in his pants.

I remember the exact moment he made the decision to commit to change. I was told that in the first part of the potty-training process it was important to let my son watch me go to the bathroom so he could see how big boys did it. So one day I grabbed him and said, "Come on, son! Let me show you what a talented guy your dad is." As I went, he stood there watching me for a moment and then suddenly started yelling, "Good boy, good boy!"

Soon afterward, he was potty trained.

Somehow that experience inspired my son to wake up to and commit to a whole new way of life. For you to throw out your old way of operating that had you stressed out, you are going to have to wake up and smell the diaper. Awakening allows you to start taking responsibility for the stress-producing circumstances that surround you and begin creating the peace you were born to have.

THE DANGERS OF STRESS ON YOUR BODY BY GOD

Stress Is the Real Deal!

Stress is not just something the advertising wizards on Madison Avenue cooked up to sell more aspirin or sleep masks filled with "magical" stress-reducing gel. It is neither a blessing nor a curse. It is not a luxury; it is not a sin.

It merely *is*. It's the "Real Deal."

Moses had it, David had it, Jesus had it, Paul had it, and if you've ever had it, then you know stress hurts. Stress is not just a term or a state of mind, it is incredibly damaging to your Body by God. Stress is something you must drastically minimize in order not to just stay sane, but to stay healthy.

The following pages in this section will help you to realize what stress does to your BBG and why you must become inspired to defend yourself against it.

Organ Alert!

Stress is created when forces *outside* the Body by God overwhelm the mind and the senses and cause a reaction in the emotional sector *inside* the Body by God.

When stress reactions occur, the resulting emotional turmoil has several very specific physical effects on the BBG's numerous organs and operating systems. Yet, unlike obviously harmful events such as a fresh cut that bleeds, the damaging and even deadly effects of stress can often be silent killers.

There is a direct link between stress and the dysfunction of various parts and systems within the BBG. Stress reactions alter the digestive system, overstimulate certain glands while *under*stimulating others, affect heart function, and change breathing. As a result, stress has an actual, measurable negative impact on blood pressure, cholesterol, electrolytes, brain chemistry, blood-sugar levels, and hormone balance.

While most people tend to look at these types of areas as normally being related to nutrition, the reality behind disease is: *"What you are eating is not nearly as important as what's eating you."* All the physiological problems associated with stress will speed up the aging process and cause or contribute to literally every type of symptom or disease known to man.

> ### Owner's Manual Recap
>
> The damaging impact of stress goes far beyond simple emotional distress. Stress also has a negative impact upon many of the physical operating systems within the BBG. Stress can not only be upsetting, but it can also produce an imbalance in body chemistry, leading to sickness and disease.

STRESS IS A SELF-INFLICTED WOUND

All BBG owners face much the same outside factors that cause stress. Work, relationships, school, personal- and family-health problems, money issues, and even positive events like weddings and parties can all be stress-producing circumstances. However, none of these things are necessarily *bad*.

Both happy events and tragedies alike cause a stress response in the body. Some stress is unavoidable. The only way to have zero stress is not to get up in the morning! On the other hand, stress becomes negative only when your *response* to it is negative. The condition we call stress is entirely *self-induced*. It is how each individual BBG owner responds to stress, and not the stress itself, that causes a negative reaction in the BBG.

Stress is not a person, a condition, or an event. Stress is a reaction to a person, a condition, or an event. Just how negative this reaction is will determine the amount of

> ### Owner's Manual Recap
>
> Whether something is stressful or not is determined by the interpretation of the individual. The level of stress and change in the emotional sector is determined by each BBG owner's reaction to outside forces—not the outside forces themselves.
>
> *See the 10 Instructions For Peace by God on page 240 for help on changing your perceptions.*

emotional turmoil and damage done to the BBG. Effectively, any injury induced by stress is a *self-inflicted wound.*

For example, public speaking can cause an undue amount of negative stress upon many BBG owners. It scares a lot of people half to death—literally. Then again, public speaking cannot be considered bad stress in and of itself, because while some people are afraid of public speaking and will suffer miserably throughout the entire experience, I and many others thoroughly enjoy speaking in public and see it as an opportunity to entertain, teach, and motivate.

REFOCUSING MY ATTENTION FROM "ME" TO "WHO ELSE" BRINGS JOY INSTEAD OF PAIN

I have faced many of the most unbearable tragedies in my life, some of which I still must confront every day. Some have left indelible footprints and scars. Nevertheless, I am still the one who chooses whether to cower and complain and let life's challenges defeat me or to stand happy, grateful, educated, and triumphant.

Anytime I am looking at life and focused on me and my problems, I become stressed and miserable. But when I choose to zero in my energy on the troubles of others, I find myself becoming energetic and motivated. Thus, I always do the best I can not to look at "me" and instead to look at "who else." "Me" is at the bottom. "Who else" is at the top.

While I am not without my moments of fear, self-pity, and regret, sooner or later I remember that the stress is not real. I eventually recall that God and others are counting on me to move and function at my best. Then my attention is back on those who need me, and the stress begins to fade.

For your own joy and for the sake of the world around you, anytime you are at the bottom thinking, *Why me?* get back on top by thinking, *Who else?*

STRESS CHANGES THE CHEMISTRY OF YOUR BODY BY GOD

One of the most destructive effects a negative stress response has within the BBG is that it alters normal internal chemistry.

The countless chemicals within the body, such as insulin, estrogen, testosterone, adrenaline, dopamine, cholesterol, and millions more regulate everything from heart rate, breathing, and digestion to thinking, moving, and even going to the bathroom.

Under normal circumstances, the cells and millions of different chemicals within the BBG have unique formulas, solutions, and molecular structures. A microscopic examination of these chemical arrangements and cells would reveal that they have a certain balance and a certain "look" to the way they are comprised. This "look" is considered "normal." This normal balance or look is present when things inside the BBG are operating properly.

However, when the effect of a negative stress response is introduced upon the BBG's many operating systems, those cells and chemicals get out of balance and actually transform. As a result, their levels and "looks" change dramatically.

For instance, the prospect of a roller-coaster ride produces varying reactions in many BBG owners. Some experience immense joy, while others experience radical fear.

Following the ride, BBG owners who enjoy roller coasters might have the exact same body chemistry as witnessed before the ride. This is due to a lack of a negative stress produced by the coaster. In fact, their BBGs may even see the addition of certain positive chemicals due to the effects of a "positive" stress response.

The BBG owners who find roller-coaster rides quite fearful, on the other hand, would have a distinctly different reaction to such stress. BBG chemicals would become imbalanced and look quite different from normal when examined after the ride was over.

This internal chemistry directly or indirectly affects and monitors every process that occurs inside the body. Therefore, the fear caused by the roller coaster or any other occurrence that causes this type of negative stress reaction does not just affect a certain chemical; it affects everything else those chemicals influence inside the BBG.

Owner's Manual Toxic-Stress Warning

Smoking, environmental pollution, toxins in household and personal hygiene items, and ingesting chemical-laden foods as discussed in the "Foods by Man" section can also directly cause something known as "chemical stress." These toxic elements stress the body's physiology and, like any stress, have a negative impact on your emotions, organ functions, and overall health.

THE STRUCTURAL EFFECTS OF STRESS

Internal factors working negatively within the BBG that are associated with stress can create many outward effects on an owner's physical makeup. Wrinkles, skin discoloration, changes in hair and nails, along with many other signs of aging can all be associated with the internal tension created by stress.

The appearance of a stressed-out BBG owner is quite distinct: hunched shoulders, bad posture, tightened muscles, and a tense expression on the face. Because structure equals function, all these elements can have harmful consequences. Constant poor spinal posture and muscle strain will speed the degenerative process and lead to pain, stiffness, joint deterioration, and even serious neurological problems.

STRESS AFFECTS THE NERVOUS SYSTEM
(YOUR BBG'S MAINFRAME COMPUTER)

When under a negative stress reaction, the sensitive nervous system sends the BBG into a virtual 911 emergency mode called "fight or flight." Fight or flight is an internal

---

Owner's Manual Physical-Stress Warning

Owners who use their Bodies by God to do manual labor or rigorous athletic activity endure *physical stress*. The body was originally created by God to hunt and gather. While physical stress can be abusive to the joints, muscles, and tendons over time, if done appropriately, it can be safe and relatively painless.

The more damaging type of physical stress is actually experienced by owners who use their BBGs to do *less* physical activities. Occupations such as accountants, cashiers, writers, lab technicians, office workers, and computer programmers who assume unnatural postures and positions all day long and are often immobile actually create the most tension on the BBG. These people are more prone to the deleterious effects of physical stress due to the chronic wrong use or lack of use of their spines, joints, ligaments, and muscles.

BBG owners with significant physical stress can compensate by following the guidelines in the Exercise by God section of the *Owner's Manual*.

alarm system created to protect the body when it is in danger. When the body is put into a state of emergency, it prepares to defend itself or run from an attack. This is done by releasing all the energy necessary to prepare for rage or sudden movement. To maximize the release of energy, this mechanism also responds by shutting or slowing down the systems designed for storing and reserving energy.

The fight-or-flight stress response releases adrenaline, causes blood to flow to the muscles and away from other organs not necessary for defense, alters the digestive process, makes glands begin to over- or undersecrete, initiates an increase in blood pressure, forces pulse and breathing rates to speed up, and triggers pupil dilation.

During sporting events, self-defense, running from a bear, or dodging a moving bullet, "fight or flight" is very helpful. However, being in this state of emergency on a regular basis is very damaging to the BBG. The constant level of excitement and overwork of the parts and systems involved in this process will eventually cause some major problems.

If the 911 stress response is elicited during times of inactivity, it is particularly hazardous. All the changes in chemical levels, organ function, and muscle tension present when the fight-or-flight mechanism is triggered are there to support some type of movement or action. If these changes are occurring while someone is neither fighting nor fleeing, but working on a computer keyboard to meet an approaching deadline, getting angry at his or her spouse, being aggravated in traffic, or upset from an irate customer's phone call, it can be extremely dangerous.

Owner's Manual Tip

When under stress, the sensitive nervous system sends the BBG into a virtual 911 emergency mode called "fight or flight." If the BBG is regularly put under stress, the organs, glands, and systems involved in this fight-or-flight response will become strained and damage themselves or cause harm in the other areas of the body that they affect.

Because the fight-or-flight mechanism is designed for action, this problem can become particularly destructive when this emergency state is induced while the body is *inactive*. This destruction is cumulative, as the damage caused by stress adds up over time.

For example: The adrenal glands respond to stress by placing more adrenaline in the bloodstream. The presence of adrenaline speeds up the function of the heart, raises blood pressure, and alters the tension of the blood vessels. All these changes in the heart are designed for an elevation in physical activity, such as running.

When excess adrenaline is put into the system without using it, there is a certain amount of injury to the heart and associated blood vessels. The level of damage increases every time this occurs, until it can eventually become fatal.

The damage caused by stress is cumulative. Each time you experience anger, resentment, worry, and fear, you create more and more destruction to the Body by God.

STRESS DEPLETES NUTRIENT STORAGE

The strain placed on the BBG during times of stress will drain essential nutritional stores that are vital to its proper function. Stress depletes vitamins, minerals, amino acids, and other important elements from the body. This will rob energy from the BBG that is necessary for the proper function of its organs and operating systems.

Nutrient energy depletion has a significant effect on the immune system. Common outward side effects of stress such as flu symptoms, cold sores, skin problems, pain, and

Owner's Manual Stressful-Eating Warning

One of the many reasons certain European countries are so much healthier than the rest of the world is not because of eating more cheese, drinking more wine, or smoking different types of cigarettes. It is cultural: Countries like France, who experience only a fraction of the heart disease that areas like America do, treat their meals with respect and as a family event. They do not regularly eat meals out of bags, inside vans, or while rushing to work.

Eating while under duress does not allow for proper digestion. The stress response changes body chemistry and the normal food assimilation process. Therefore, food is not broken down and has the potential to be left in places like your arteries.

NOTE: Follow the guidelines in the Food by God section to help avoid some of the health problems inherent with stressful eating.

illness are all evidence of how stress can suppress the immune system. A weakened immune system can lead to less-obvious developments of internal illness, such as cancer and autoimmune diseases.

With all the negative effects the body endures when in a state of anxiety, immune-system defense is needed more than ever. Yet, in fact, just the opposite is taking place: When stressed, the immune system is weakened, putting the entire BBG in an extremely vulnerable state.

If your life is a hard pill to swallow, swallowing good food and vitamins may be doing you no good. Again, *what you are eating is not nearly as important as what is eating you.*

17 | ARE YOU PROGRAMMED FOR STRESS?

The way you look at the world you live in has, in many ways, been programmed.
This programming can, however, be uninstalled and upgraded.

Learning to deprogram or reprogram yourself from feeling the effects and triggers of stress will save you from much of the serious physical damage stress can cause and drastically improve your life. This section will show you how to clear up your internal hard drive, thus leaving you plenty of room to download newer and better files and feel the peace you are lacking in your life.

Here is where we start . . .

SEEING THE WORLD THROUGH YOUR "PERCEPTION SOFTWARE"

Freud, Spock, Jung, and Einstein might argue, but in many ways your emotions have been *programmed* into you, just like a computer.

You have "Perception Software" that has been downloaded into you throughout your life and that determines how you *see* the world. Perception is nine-tenths of the law. In most cases, it is your *point of view* of people, issues, and events and not the people, issues, and events themselves that determines how you react to them, define them, and create your version of the story.

Your Perception Software has programmed your point of view, which will ultimately determine your emotional responses. Most everyone looks at life's circumstances differently. Different people look at the same incident and, due to their different perceptions, report completely different versions. What happened, who's at fault, and almost every other detail will vary from person to person.

It is your *perceptions* that often will decide whether something is positive or negative to you. Some people see a challenge or conflict as an overwhelming problem, some see the same scenarios as small, and some do not see them as problems at all.

This viewpoint programming will determine how swiftly and confidently you act and on what scale you measure the issues that affect your life. It will influence your expectations of people, how you manage controversy, how you judge and treat others, and how you handle relationships in the different areas of your life.

In many ways, your programming will determine your success in life. If you put someone with a poverty mind-set in a wealthy area, they will find a way to live in poverty. On the contrary, if you put someone with a wealthy mind-set in an impoverished area, they will soon own half the real estate and be renting it out to the people with the poverty mind-sets.

Types of Perception Software

Your Perception Software can be generalized to fit into several basic areas:

History Software. Your experience with certain circumstances, people, events, conflicts, and education make up your History Software. These past experiences will often totally determine how you feel about every new experience.

- If you have a "history" of dealing with complex or uncertain events like a flat tire or a stock market crash, then you know what to do and you have some idea how it turns out. As a result, your history programming allows you to more easily handle the situation and be less stressed.
- If you have never had children, then when you are eating dinner in a restaurant, flying on an airplane, or sitting in a movie theater and someone has a crying baby or a disruptive child, you are not programmed to understand. As a result, your

programming may make you become completely intolerant to the noise or behavior. However, if you have children, you already know what the experience is like. While you may not be thrilled to listen to a child cry during the movie or while you are trying to eat, or even sleep on the plane, your History Software tells you to show some compassion.

Cultural Software. Your mother, father, siblings, occupation, peer group, geographic area, school, or religion together or individually make up your Cultural Software.

Different cultures put tremendous importance on certain ideas and have very specific ways, rules, and in some cases, strict laws on how people should behave, work, and treat others.

Goal Software. The intensity of the desire you have to obtain all your wants and needs will make up your Goal Software.

The level of your desire to obtain wealth, meet needs, be on time, find perfection, and the intensity at which you pursue ethical or religious standards and ideals will determine the effects of your Goal Software on your perceptions.

- People meticulous about every detail being perfect and all things being in order have Goal Software that has programmed them for severe inner turmoil from something as simple as a typo on a page, a disorderly desk, or a messy kitchen.

Cultural Software Affects How You See Yourself, Judge Yourself, and See and Judge Others

- If the culture you grew up in believes that good people wear only black hats, dress in green clothes, eat blue food, and should be accountants, you will be programmed to think that anyone who wears a red hat, dresses in yellow clothes, eats pink food, or is a fireman is bad.
- As I mentioned earlier, my family grew up in New York City. The tendency is for people in that culture not to openly express love, to be fast to judge, to be cynical, and to have high and unrealistic expectations of others. The world-famous "New York attitude" is really a result of cultural programming.

On the other hand, others who are not programmed this way will feel little or no stress at all in the same situations.

Self-Esteem Software. How you see yourself and how you feel others see you make up your Self-Esteem Software. How you envision yourself will massively influence what future you feel you are capable of attaining and how you will interact with others. Your Self-Esteem Software can therefore determine whether or not you will go to college, what college you will attend, what courses you will take, what occupation you will choose, and whom you will decide to marry.

- The key to experiencing good relationships in your life is typically not based on the performance of the other person in it. It is your Self-Esteem Software, which programs your own confidence and feelings of worthiness, that will be the greatest determining factor in how well you relate to others.

> **Self-Esteem and Goal Software are massively influenced by History and Cultural Software.**

SEEING THE WORLD THROUGH YOUR OWN SET OF GLASSES (OR CALLING 'EM LIKE YOU SEE 'EM!)

Things are not absolutely negative or absolutely positive, black or white, yellow or red. How you *see* things depends on what kind of glasses you are wearing.

The only time you are injured by what appear to be stressful times and events in your life is when you begin to feel overpowered by them. When the glasses you are looking through *see* that you are a victim of stress, that is the only time stress is necessarily bad. When you see your problems as being in control of your emotions, health, and success, that is the only time when the physical and mental damage of stress applies.

It is the final inning of the final game in the World Series, and the score is tied. The bases are loaded, there are two outs, and the final batter now has three balls and two strikes. The next pitch will most likely decide the game and the Series. The final pitch is thrown, the batter does not swing, and the catcher is holding on to the ball. You can hear a pin drop in the sold-out stadium as everyone waits for the umpire to make the call.

When he doesn't say anything, a fan finally screams, "Well, what is it?"

The umpire says, "It ain't nothing until I call it."

It isn't stress until you call it stress; and you call 'em like you see 'em.

For your world to improve and your stress to be reduced, you must begin *seeing* life through a totally different pair of glasses from those you are used to wearing, or at least start changing the prescription for your lenses. To change your prescription, you must change your perception software.

Deleting the Prejudice of Programming

Understanding your Perception Software should help you begin to understand others' as well. We all come from different places. We all have different programming based on our life experiences. There is a saying: "If you were them, you would act exactly the same way." This means that if someone is handling issues or behaving in a manner you do not agree with, if you had similar Perception Programming, you would respond and behave in the same manner. You would *see* the world as that person *sees* it.

All our perceptions are *limited* to what we have encountered in life. When you develop a viewpoint based on *limited* knowledge, it is called a "prejudice."

Prejudice is defined as "an opinion formed without adequate reason or substantial information—usually negative."

All our words and actions are *limited* by our different Perception Software. We are all drastically influenced by how each of us is programmed to see the world. By understanding this, hopefully you can delete your prejudices and improve your reactions to other people and events.

Deleting prejudice programming means making an effort to understand where other people are coming from and gaining more knowledge about other individuals, professions, groups, organizations, and circumstances before forming an opinion or making a judgment about them. That is a more heavenly perception: *"Even God waits until the end before judging."*

Downloading, Deleting, and Reprogramming
Perception Software (You Are an "Upgrade" in Progress)

In all areas of your life, some of your greatest limitations to success are the walls your perceptions build around you. If you examine your life carefully, as you should each day, quite frequently you should come to the conclusion that certain areas are not working out as they should, and that some of the things you do don't make sense.

When I look at kids wearing pants around their knees, poking holes all over their bodies, depressed over a lack of popularity, taking drugs, dropping out of school, or doing all sorts of tragic things with their lives, I realize that they are just working off the wrong *software*. Something about their histories, the culture around them, and/or their self-esteem has *programmed* them to think that some terrible things, awful goals, and the need to be accepted by teenagers, or be in love at sixteen, actually "make sense."

As adults, we are often not much different. We live in a world where our health, our finances, our emotional states, our families, and our planet's peace are in constant turmoil. Yet, very few people ever change their courses. Many have become programmed to take pills rather than change their health, to accept limited financial resources and depression rather than change their views and occupation, to get married and divorced too easily, and to blame others for our wars rather than looking in the mirror at our own internal wars first.

In order to see a change in your life, you must change the way you are programmed. You must begin to identify the Perception Software that must be deleted and what must be downloaded in order for you to go to the next level.

Being weaned on the "New York attitude" culture created an incredible amount of stress in my life. Interacting with others who judged me solely on my performance and didn't love me just for me caused me to have low self-esteem, be nervous about performing well, and become a neurotic, overachieving workaholic. Nonetheless, rather than blaming a culture, my geography, or my family for my stress, I have worked to examine and recognize my programming, delete it, and download better files.

All your Perception Software issues *can* be fixed. While deleting and downloading new software may be more difficult to do on a person than on a computer, due to all of our hard-drive (head) problems, the reality is that you *can* be reprogrammed.

Reprogramming takes looking at the world from a totally different place and angle than you have ever looked at it before. It takes continually examining your thoughts, emotions, and reactions and determining where they came from. Once you have identified the source of your programming and that your reactions are in fact programmed, you can begin to work on deleting the faulty programming and downloading more positive, peaceful files.

Only God has the maximum necessary upgrade. You, on the other hand, are an *upgrade in progress.* By working on *"The 10 Instructions for Peace by God"* to follow and *waking up* to being reprogrammed, you will begin to create more peace by downloading new software from heaven.

Owner's Manual Tip

See the Time by God section to learn how to fit reprogramming your Perception Software into your busy schedule.

18 | OWNER'S MANUAL GUIDELINES FOR STRESS MANAGEMENT

10 Instructions for Peace by God

There is no such thing as "poverty management" or "disease management." If you are broke or diseased, that is hard or downright impossible to manage. There is, however, such a thing as financial management or health management. By appropriately managing your finances and your health, you work to avoid the pain of poverty and disease.

It is the same with stress. You do not manage your stress; you manage your peace. Peace is the normal, natural state God created. Not stress. If your life activities, your outlook, and your relationships are causing fear, depression, and anxiety to rage out of control, the bottom line is, that is stressful. It is very difficult to manage stress. God created you to manage peace.

Peace is not something you find when your latest crisis is over. What usually follows stress, of course, is the *next stress*. Peace is not discovered; it is created.

You don't make *less stress*, you create more peace. Creating peace does not begin by changing everyone and all the situations that surround you. Changing locations, jobs, or spouses is typically *not* the answer. While the grass always seems greener (more peaceful) in someone else's yard, occupation, or relationship, once you get over there, over there becomes over here again.

As the adage says, "Wherever you go, there you are." Start with yourself. If you want to see your environment and the people around you change, the best way for that to happen is for *you* to change first.

It is easy to blame circumstances for your stress. The problem with that philosophy is that when you blame things outside yourself for your troubles, this creates a self-defeating outlook on life. You believe that *nothing* can be done to overcome. You also put the power of your life outside you when it is truly inside you.

The real roots of your stress come from within. It is the way you look at and administrate your life that causes most of your pain and aggravation. That is okay. It is actually *great news!* The easiest thing in the world to change is *you*. People can be tough to change, and family, jobs, and situations may even be impossible to change. But you can change right here, right now. Working on *you* is wealth and health management, not poverty and disease management.

It is *peace management*, not stress management.

To build or create anything, you must follow the instructions. To create peace, follow "The 10 Instructions for Peace by God," and get ready to receive downloads from heaven.

These 10 Instructions for Peace by God are the ideal way to act and look at the world so you can be reprogrammed and significantly reduce negative stress. Like most ideals, they are something you constantly strive for, but most likely will never totally obtain.

When I first wrote this list, I asked my wife, Dr. Sheri, to look it over for me. Rather than making suggestions or pointing out grammatical errors, she just circled which ones I wasn't doing.

Like you, I am also an "upgrade and a work in progress."

The 10 Instructions

1. Thou Shalt Be Appearanceless
2. Thou Shalt Be Wantless
3. Thou Shalt Be Acceptanceless
4. Thou Shalt Be Resultless
5. Thou Shalt Be Prideless
6. Thou Shalt Be Timeless
7. Thou Shalt Be Hateless
8. Thou Shalt Be Fearless
9. Thou Shalt Be Faithful
10. Thou Shalt Be Hopeful

INSTRUCTION #1: THOU SHALT BE APPEARANCELESS

There Is No Peace in a Life Spent Wishing You Were What You Are Not

Our infatuation with appearance will never lead us down a smooth and peaceful path. If you rely on how you look to decide how you feel, you will always be a zit or a bad hair day away from misery. Beauty is totally unreliable; it is a fact of life. You cannot count on it from one day or one decade to the next. Yet, from just before puberty on, people spend endless hours and countless dollars on improving how they look.

It is not a bad thing to always try to look your best. But when you allow your appearance to determine who you are, how you feel about yourself, your health, or how successful you can become, you are limiting yourself and tying on to a very fragile, shaky foundation. Being too concerned about appearance means setting yourself up for a life full of stress, illness, and many falls from grace.

When I was in elementary school they always took a class picture at the end of every year. In these pictures, the tallest kids were in the back row, and the shortest were in the front. I started out in kindergarten toward the tall row, but by the second grade, I had made my way all the way down to the very front. In fact, eventually, I was not only in the front, I was front and center, where only the shortest of the short reside.

In addition to being vertically challenged, I had a large, curly red afro, freckles from forehead to toe, and my parents apparently enjoyed the color plaid. To say the least, I was considered a bit peculiar, and often found myself being chosen last for all the teams in gym class and had trouble with anything requiring the need to be picked as a partner.

As years went by, things slowly improved, and I eventually recognized the need for more regular haircuts, sunscreen, and wearing solid colors. Unfortunately, the bottom line was that I was still very different from my classmates. Clothing and better hairstyles could not cover up the fact that I was a short guy with red hair who was mentally and emotionally traumatized from growing up as an outcast. As a result of all my peculiarities, I spent the majority of my early life wishing I were somebody else.

For years, I wished I was not so different. I wanted to be taller, have better hair, a cooler personality, and parents with different genes—and better taste in clothes. Then, suddenly, something happened that began to lessen my desire to be different.

I had a son.

Luckily for my little boy, Skylar, he has good hair, and unlike my parents, I don't like plaid. He came out beautiful, charming, and well dressed. The reality is, however, that regardless of what he would have looked or acted like, I would have loved him just the same. In fact, if he were physically or emotionally challenged in some way that would have made life harder for him, my heart would have gone out to him even more. I eventually realized that a father's love surpasses all appearances.

Of far greater importance than what my son looks like is who he really is. When it comes to my son, I look right through what other people see. I see what they do not see, and I love what he looks like no matter what.

Today, I no longer feel peculiar; I feel special. I know that when my Father-God looks at me, He loves what He has created. He loves what He sees, even when I have a zit or a bad hair day. Knowing that, I don't wish I were someone else anymore. I am now much more *appearanceless* (although, sometimes, I wouldn't mind being just a little bit taller).

I always do all I can at the time to look my best, but I really try not to allow what I look like to determine who I am or what I feel like.

When you are too caught up in how you look, you also tend to get too caught up in how *others* look. Of equal importance to not judging your own appearance too harshly is not judging the appearance of others. Just as our Father-God looks past your face in deciding how He feels about you, so should you look past the faces of others. When it is said, "Do not judge a book (or person) by the cover," it really means to be appearanceless—with others as well as yourself.

> The LORD said . . . , "Do not consider his appearance or his height [be appearanceless], for I have rejected him. The LORD does not look at the things man looks at. Man looks at the outward appearance, but the LORD looks at the heart." (1 Sam. 16:7)

The River of Dreams: The Peace of Appearanceless

An old legend tells of a river that exists high up on a mountain and deep in the forest called the "River of Dreams." As in most legends, finding this mystical river is very difficult, and the journey there is extremely hazardous. Despite that fact, countless men and women have been willing to sacrifice years of their lives and have even died attempting to discover it. The reason so many feel the River of Dreams is worth the risk is that the legend states if you stand in its waters and gaze down into your reflection, you will see all you desire yourself to be.

If you wish for good looks, you will see beauty. If you want to have athletic ability, you will see yourself soaring over the highest bar, kicking the winning goal, or crossing the line first for the gold medal. If you seek health, you will witness complete and total vitality. And if you wish to be popular, you will instantly be looking upon a picture of yourself surrounded by hundreds of admirers, all attentive to your every word.

Most who seek the River of Dreams never find it. Tragically, those who do discover these tempting waters rarely leave it. Once seeing a vision of themselves as they always wished they were, they cannot turn back and face their own reality. They become doomed to a life of staring into the water, lost in an illusion for all eternity.

It is said that only those who truly have Peace by God will be able to escape the River of Dreams. This is because when they step into it and look down at their reflection, they see themselves exactly as they already are.

They are *appearanceless*.

INSTRUCTION #2: THOU SHALT BE WANTLESS

If You Want Nothing, Nothing Can Be Taken from You

The first verse in Psalm 23 says, "The LORD is my shepherd, I shall not be in want." *Not to want* is some exceptionally good advice. Unfortunately, not to be in want is not to be human.

Your BBG was literally *born* wanting. The dilemma begins when you go from just wanting food and a dry diaper to wanting a nicer car, a bigger home, a different job, a better body, a larger bank account, a tropical vacation, and the latest electronic gadget. As you begin to desire more and more, what you desire begins to drive your thoughts, control your actions, and determine the direction you and your emotions are going. When you start to decide how you are doing by how much you have of what you want or how close you are to getting it, you have become a slave to your wants. Ultimately, your wants become your masters and your shepherds.

To continue to create peace, you must learn to become both ambitious *and* content.

Set goals and always strive to have more, but be happy with what you already possess. Have wants, but also be WANTLESS.

Remember, you can't work your way into heaven. Constantly seeking more will often cause you to look past what is truly important. If you believe you must reach your goals to be worthy or satisfied with life, you will rarely, if ever, find peace. *Being a miserable achiever is practically a proverb.*

Perhaps the most universal thing people *think* they want is financial freedom, because they believe money will bring them peace. The problem is, there is no such thing as financial freedom. If you do not have money, you worry about where you are going to get it. If you *have* it, you worry about it being taken away. The bottom line is, if you want money, you are going to worry about money.

Like money, the tragedy of getting what you want is that it never really ends up being truly fulfilling, and it almost never satisfies the want. Cars get old, gadgets get broken, and vacations end. Acquisitions rarely bring lasting joy and usually bring with them even more concern about money.

When I want something badly and I believe life will be really good once I get it, I have found that no matter how noble or worthy that want may be, I usually experience a large amount of stress and frustration—and get only a small amount of sleep. It is only after I decide all I really want is for God's will to be done that I can just sit back, do what He puts right there in front me, relax, and patiently wait for it to happen.

The really tough nights are when I allow my mind to race around, worrying about not getting what I want or having the wants that I already possess taken from me. It is only after making the decision to let all my wants go that I finally get some rest.

Nothing can be taken from me when I want nothing. When I am no longer a slave to the wants in my life, I begin to determine my own direction. When God, and not a want, is my Master or my "Shepherd," I trust I am being given whatever I actually need. While I may not get the fleeting things I want, I am getting everything God wants for me.

If you want nothing, then nothing can be taken from you. Everything you want can be taken from you, but nothing can be taken that God wants you to have. Only what God gives you is truly money in the bank!

The Shepherd Tenet

A shepherd guides his sheep toward the place he knows will bring them food, comfort, security, and safety. His role in life is to keep and protect the flock and look after their well-being at all times. If they stray, he finds them and brings them back to the fold. If they are hurt, he sees that they are healed. If they are in danger, he himself fights off the predator or removes the sheep from harm's way.

The sheep must trust the shepherd to do all these things. Like a baby sleeping safely in his crib or a child riding comfortably in the backseat of a car, the sheep have total faith that their needs are always going to be met. They are not concerned about the place they are in life, as they trust they are exactly where they should be. They blindly follow the shepherd, innocently believe they are headed in the right direction, and trust they will get to their destination precisely on time.

You can startle sheep, but peace always returns to the flock. They fear no evil, for they know the shepherd is with them. Even in the presence of their enemies his rod and his staff comfort them.

Being not just led, but herded, by God—the Shepherd—has the capacity to bring total peace and joy to your life. All the 10 Instructions can be found in the Shepherd Tenet. Follow Him like a sheep, and "surely goodness and love will follow [you] all the days of [your] life" (Ps. 23:6).

The Shepherd's Tenet

To want only what God wants to give you, and trust that He will give you everything you need—and more than you ever wanted.

Live for the Mission and Want Nothing Else . . . and Get All You Want!

Life's mission is to serve God, care for others, and build and rebuild yourself. Living for the mission—and not for what you want—is your best chance to get what you want.

- If you want better health, don't focus on illness, focus on the activities of achieving better health.
- If you want more loving, committed relationships, don't focus on loneliness and strife; focus on being more loving and being more committed.
- If you want more success in your work, don't focus on failure, focus on perfecting your skills, learning new skills, and improving your work habits.

Be *wantless* and get all you want!

INSTRUCTION #3: THOU SHALT BE ACCEPTANCELESS

Do What Is Right, Not What Is Acceptable

Today, if your looks, actions, beliefs, possessions, personality, and favorite TV show match up with what the people around you like or believe in, you are accepted. Tomorrow, if you change any of these things or if those around you change, you are no longer accepted.

The bottom line is that people tend to like you only if *you* like what *they* like. Especially if you like *them*. This works fine, unless, of course, you think, look, or act differently or accidentally insult them.

Then they don't like you anymore . . .

Acceptance of others is biased, fleeting, and often holds no real reason or value. That is why if you are seeking acceptance, you will often be without peace. Just look at athletes and ninth-grade physics geniuses. The athlete has acceptance, but it will be gone as soon as his career ends or his talent wanes. The ninth-grade physics genius won't be accepted until he's graduated from college with his Ph.D. and helps put the first man on Pluto.

The acceptance of man is not real. It is a fleeting ghost that can appear or disappear at any moment.

Opinions are like noses. Everyone's got one—and they smell. The views of the people who surround you are always limited in some way, and so are automatically prone to prejudice. It is human nature to allow these viewpoints to exclude or look down upon other people. Being a crowd-pleaser and choosing jobs, classes, attitudes, and lifestyles that are accepted by others and not desired by you is legendary for creating failure.

The desire for acceptance has caused kids to steal candy, teenagers to take drugs, smoke, drink, and commit suicide, and adults to end up in a place that has left them impoverished and in despair.

Just because something *is* popular doesn't make it right, and just because something is *not* popular doesn't make it wrong. Settling on who you think you are or who you think the people around you are, based on popular opinion, is wrong. It may sometimes make others like you, but it will rarely make *you* like you. If you are looking for acceptance, you will often see yourself as less than you really are.

Don't believe in ghosts! Stop doing what other people believe you should do, and begin doing what you believe you should do. *Do what is right, not what is acceptable.* Others may not always like you, but *you* will like you.

Consensus as a whole is usually blind. Following the crowd will cause you to walk into walls, puddles, and busy intersections. Rarely will the crowd lead you toward peace. Be *acceptanceless.* Do not follow the blind.

Instead, lead them.

> Be imitators of God . . . I urge you to live a life worthy of the calling you have received. (Eph. 5:1; 4:1)

Developing Standards of Integrity: Becoming a Mirror for God

In order to become completely "free from the need for acceptance," you must discover who you really are and what you should be like. Once you understand what are good and proper goals for your life and your behavior, you can stop following the crowd and begin following your heart.

There is truly only one "right" way to act. Act like God. You are not God, but you can try to copy Him. In your life, try to behave as if you are a mirror held up in front of God. Then attempt to let everything you say and do be a *reflection* of His qualities:

- Be completely humble and gentle; be patient, bearing with one another in love (Eph. 4:2).
- Make every effort to add to your faith goodness; and to goodness, knowledge; and to knowledge, self-control; and to self-control, perseverance; and to perseverance, godliness; and to godliness, brotherly kindness; and to brotherly kindness, love. (2 Peter 1:5–7)
- Whatever is true, whatever is noble, whatever is right, whatever is pure, whatever is lovely, whatever is admirable—if anything is excellent or praiseworthy—think about such things . . . Put it into practice. And the God of peace will be with you. (Phil. 4:8–9)

Qualities of God List

Humbleness, Gentleness, Patience, Love, Faithfulness, Goodness, Knowledge, Self-Control, Perseverance, Godliness, Brotherly Kindness, Truthfulness, Nobleness, Rightness, Purity, Loveliness, Admirability, Excellence, Praiseworthiness, Peacefulness.

When someone judges or criticizes you, if the suggestion is on the "Qualities of God List," heed it. If it didn't make the list, ignore it. Choosing to mirror God rather than mirror the crowd is called *integrity*. By living with integrity and standing by godly properties, no matter *what*, you may not always be popular or successful in the short run, but integrity always wins out and gains the trust and respect of others in the long run.

The integrity of the upright guides them. (Prov. 11:3)

Regifting Criticism and Praise

Jesus said, *"I don't accept praise from men,"* *(John 5:41).* This is because Jesus knows it is the nature of men for their acceptance to be conditional, temporary, and based on limited wisdom.

I once was visiting a friend's house right after my birthday. He told me that he forgot to get me anything, but that I could take whatever I wanted from the "regift closet." The "regift closet" was a towel closet by his guest bathroom that contained all the gifts he had received over the years that he didn't ask for, didn't like, and didn't want. On holidays, special occasions, or incidences where he had forgotten someone's birthday, he gave out these gifts. Thus the term "regift."

You can do the same thing with judgment that does not come from God. When someone offers you criticism that you didn't ask for and don't like, it is yours only if you accept it. Actually, if you do not accept a gift at all from someone, then whose is it? It is still really the other person's. In this way, the criticism is instantly regifted back to the person who offered it.

Thus, if someone were to criticize you, you would not feel discouraged. If someone were to praise you, you would not feel proud. You should actually take both criticism and praise the same way. So if someone tells you that you are great OR if someone tells you that you stink and your mother wears army boots, you should look at both comments similarly. You do not accept either one (unless, of course, you have not showered or your mother requires some significant fashion advice). Praise and criticism are not necessarily bad. They become a problem only if you allow what others believe you are to become who you believe you are.

Peace will not come if what others think or say about you becomes what you think or say about yourself. Jesus knew this, and so would not seek or accept acceptance from men, only from God. God's opinion is not temporary or limited in any way.

While it is important to have good, trusted teachers, coaches, and mentors around you at all times to help you grow and prosper, pick the opinions you value very carefully. If you are relatively sure of how God wishes you to behave and proceed with your life, you will need very little input or comment from others. You will undoubtedly get it, but you usually will not need it.

Jesus did not accept praise or criticism from men, because both may be gifts without value.

> I do not accept praise from men, but I know you. I know that you do not have the love of God in your hearts. (John 5:41–42)
>
> Or, in other words: I'm rubber; you're glue. Whatever you say bounces off me and sticks to you.

INSTRUCTION #4: THOU SHALT BE RESULTLESS

In the Game of Life, It's Far Better to Be "1 and 20" than "0 and 0"

If a professional baseball player gets only one hit out of every three times he bats, he's an all-star. In other words, if he fails twice as often as he succeeds, he is still considered one of the best baseball players in the world. Even more, if he were to fail as often as he succeeds, get one hit out of every two at bats, they would name the stadium, the airport, and half the roads in the city after him!

If a professional baseball player could only enjoy the game when he *wins*, he'd hate playing nearly *all* the time. Peace cannot be created while focusing only on the results of your efforts. The reality to the game of life is that you are going to strike out once in a while. You are going to lose some games, possibly more than you will win. If your peace of mind is dependent only on your results, you are going to be stressed as often as you are not—or maybe even more often.

If a doctor, lawyer, coach, salesman, teacher, or athlete is only happy when he wins, or when other people are appreciative of him, he will live a roller-coaster life of highs, lows, and frequent breakdowns. If you can be content only with victory, life is going to be a long and painful season.

To begin enjoying *all* of life more, you have to detach yourself from results. In order to do this, you have to pay more attention to enjoying just playing the game and less attention to how it turns out. When you do this you become *resultless*. A resultless life is a lot more fun and a lot less stressful. Most childhood competitions understand this: You get an award just for participating.

Owner's Manual Warning: Do Not Try This at Home!

Although you may build the peace and confidence necessary to not need or accept praise, others around you still do. Do not withhold praise from your wife, husband, children, coworkers, barber, or grocery store clerk. In fact, overpraise whenever possible. Trust me on this one.

Also, in addition to being acceptanceless, like Jesus, you must be accepting.

Consequences

Whenever you think of *consequences*, you almost always think of bad ones, right? Rarely do you think, *What happens if I succeed?* Instead, you think: *What if I strike out? What if I miss? What if I fall? What if I make a mistake? What if I fail? What if I . . ."*

Because of the fear of consequences, you end up being so cautious and playing so badly, you usually end up creating the very consequences you feared in the first place. Ironically, because you fear missing, falling, or making a mistake, you miss, fall, and make a mistake. The ultimate tragedy to fearing is that it may become so great that you do not even get in the game at all.

I have watched many of the best Olympic, professional, and amateur athletes I have ever worked with go into competition and lose because of the fear of consequences. Often, winning comes down to more than ability; it comes down to a change in the *consequences*.

The athletes I have seen win the most medals and championships were not always the best, but the ones who thought of good consequences. They thought, *What if I hit it? What if I make it? What if I score a 10? What if they love me?* or *What if I win?* It is the athletes who wanted to get up to the plate with two outs in the last inning, who looked to take the last shot of the game, and who sought the opportunity to step into the arena with every eye focused on them who have made history and revealed their greatness.

People who perform without thinking of the consequences and just "go for it," are the ones who have the best chance of winning. If they lose, at least they gave it their best shot and can live their life without regrets.

Rather than thinking about consequences, think, *What would I do if I knew I could not fail?*

When the score is taken at the end of your life, let it be said that you won some and lost some. But don't let it be said that you never even came off the bench. *Sometimes, all that matters in life is forgetting the consequences and going for it.*

It is far better to be 1 and 20, than 0 and 0.

See Rule #4: "Inspired to Win" of "The Four Rules of Olympic Success" on page 27 for more information on overcoming "Consequences."

Joseph Had Only a 1 and 3 Record, but Wound Up in the Bible Hall of Fame

The story of Joseph (Gen. 37–50) is a story of *resultlessness*. God shows us through Joseph that you should not worry about the results of a single game, but how the entire season turns out.

Like all of us, Joseph was given gifts and talents by God. When Joseph took his abilities on the road, he couldn't put a single point in the win column. At first, Joseph suffered nothing but one-sided losses. Nonetheless, because Joseph had faith and trusted in God's overall plan, he was able to look past his winless streak and bring victory for millions.

Due to the famine, Joseph's brothers went to Egypt to get food. At that point, Joseph had a perfect opportunity for mockery, hatred, and revenge. However, as a courageous overcomer of losses who understood the divine will of God, Joseph fed his brothers and made one of the most significant statements in the entire Bible. Joseph said, "Don't be afraid. Am I in the place of God? You intended to harm me, but God intended it for good to accomplish what is now being done, the saving of many lives" (Gen. 50:19–20).

Joseph lost three times as often as he won, *but God was undefeated.* Even with only a 1 and 3 overall record, Joseph ended up in the Bible Hall of Fame.

The Career of Joseph:

1 Win, 3 Losses—a .250 Winning Percentage

- Loss: Joseph, at a tender and young age, was cast into a pit by his own brothers.
- Loss: Later, wishing to make a profit off him, Joseph's brothers sold him into slavery in Egypt.
- Loss: Potiphar's wife tried to lure Joseph into committing adultery. Not wanting to perform this horrible sin against God, he defied her. Feeling scorned, Potiphar's wife had Joseph arrested on rape charges and locked away in prison.
- Win: Joseph was made the highest official in the king's court and overseer of all Egypt. Using the ability God gave him to interpret dreams, Joseph saved Egypt and the surrounding nations from a famine that would have cost countless lives.

Loss Is Often Opportunity in Disguise

God has a purpose for everything under the sun. All things, even losses, can be used for His good. The history books are jam-packed with people who were terribly injured, went bankrupt, had someone they loved die, and/or lost time and time again, but who used their immense defeats to create incredible victories. While losses may at first *appear* to be failures, often they become God's road signs, leading us in the direction we need to go so that He wins BIG.

God never loses. He is "infinity and 0."

You can look at many trials in your life and wonder why God does not let you off the hook. You can look at many people and be angry at them for the turmoil they create in your life. Yet, the truth is, it may be God's will that you are handed these losses. There is no one person or incident you should hate or begrudge. The things that come against you and cause your defeats may be the actual instruments God is using to put you in a place where you can do His work—and win.

It is often within the hurt and the storm that God turns your heart and your focus in the proper direction. Losses are often the defining moments in your life that decide if you are worthy and courageous enough to answer God's call, or if you will cower and be crushed. Just as in the life of Joseph, *loss is often an opportunity in disguise*, an opportunity to save lives and bring ultimate victory for God.

> **A lot of people ask God to help them stop losing,
> only to find out it is God who is creating the losses.**

Happiness Is: Staying Focused on Your Mission, Not Your Results

The Happiness Equation states: If your reality in life meets or exceeds your expectations of life, you will be happy. But if your expectations are too great, you will be unhappy. The more overblown your expectations, the unhappier you will be.

The Happiness Equation

$$\text{Happiness} = \frac{\text{Reality}}{\text{Expectation}}$$

Example Equations

Expectation: At 9:00 A.M., I am going to get hit over the head.
Reality: At 9:00 A.M., I didn't get hit over the head.
   =Happy/Thrilled (Reality exceeded expectations)

Expectation: I don't think people should get hit over the head with an eggbeater.
Reality: At 9:00 a.m., you are hit over the head with an eggbeater.
   =Misery (Reality did not meet or exceed expectations)

Expectation: The only car worth driving is a brand-new Ferrari.
Reality: You drive an old Pinto.
   =Misery

Expectation: I just want a vehicle that works and gets me from point A to point B.
Reality: You drive an old Pinto (that works).
   =Happiness

For example: If you expect to be able to wake up in the morning and not have someone beat you over the head with an eggbeater, but the reality is that every day for five years I have shown up at your house at 9:00 A.M. beat you over the head with an eggbeater, you will *not* be happy.

However, if one day at 9:00 A.M. I do *not* show up, according to the Happiness Equation, you *will* be happy. In fact, in this case, your reality *exceeds* your expectations. After five years of getting beaten with an eggbeater every morning, you are actually *expecting* it. Thus, you will not only be happy, you will be *thrilled*.

I have done a lot of peace management training for teachers. These incredible men and women became teachers because they truly felt a mission to work with children. They all had expectations that nothing but joy could come from a mission of helping kids learn, grow, overcome family disharmony, and have a better chance at a successful future. Unfortunately, as a whole, these groups were without a doubt some of the most unhappy, stressed-out people I have ever worked with. The stress and unhappiness hits them hardest when they lose focus on their mission and instead develop expectations of *results* that exceed a teacher's reality.

The Happiness Equation explains this perfectly . . .

Example Equations for Teachers

Expectation: To reach every child.
Reality: On any given day or year, some kids may be extremely difficult or impossible to reach.

Expectation: Typical occupational challenges.
Reality: Parents, broken homes, and school systems offer much greater challenges than a typical job.

Expectation: Contentment with only what a teacher's salary can afford.
Reality: Desire for better homes, cars, and more financial security.

The result of each of these equations = unhappiness. In each and every case, expectation exceeds reality.

Teachers have an awesome mission. They have an opportunity to affect the lives of thousands of children over the span of their careers. Each child is incredibly valuable and precious to God. If teachers could stay focused on the expectation that, in their mission, making a difference in even just one life is a gigantic thing, then they would stay happy.

I was nineteen years old before the first teacher finally broke through my thick skull. However, the reality was that dozens of teachers had made little dents and paved the way. Some planted, some watered, and finally some reaped a harvest. Each one of my teachers who cared and reached out to me took part in giving me hope and a future. I gave most of them a really difficult time, but if they all had known and stayed focused on the end result, they would have been more likely to enjoy working with a young monster like me.

Sadly, it is so easy to lose sight of your mission. Eventually, rather than our expectations being "to make a difference," many of us begin wanting more results than what our personal realities have to offer. We get lost in immense challenges we were not expecting, but which are the reality of our lives or professions. The end result of our equation is misery.

I have worked with many patients who are eighty, ninety, or over a hundred years old who are still extremely healthy. One of the most amazing things I see with these folks is that they tend to have a peaceful attitude. You can see it on their faces. You can read it in their expressions.

One of my more healthy, positive octogenarians once told me, "If I am still pumping blood and sucking air, then it is a good day!" Now *that's* an expectation (result) that is *not* too hard to exceed. With *that* mission, your life will always equal happiness—literally—until the day you die.

Resultless = Happiness.

Owner's Manual Happiness-While-Wanting-More Tip

You can still want more and find happiness. All you have to do while doing what it takes to get more is be content with who and where you are.

INSTRUCTION #5: THOU SHALT BE PRIDELESS

GOD, me (BIG GOD, little me)

A young associate pastor at a Midwestern, old-fashioned church impatiently waited for his opportunity to stand before the pulpit to preach and bring the church to the next level. He knew he had better ideas, superior speaking skills, and a more dynamic presentation than the senior pastor. He believed if he could just get the chance, he had the charisma to really save some souls, increase the attendance numbers, and blow the roof off the church.

One Sunday, the senior pastor was called out of town on a family emergency. The young pastor was elated that he was finally going to get the opportunity to lead the congregation. He stepped confidently up to the pulpit and immediately began to scream about repentance, quote Scriptures from memory, and tell the stories he had created.

About halfway through the sermon, he noticed the back two rows begin to clear out. Frustrated, he began to scream even louder and hit the congregation with more severe fire and brimstone. When he noticed some people at the sides beginning to nod off to sleep, he even began jumping up and down, in one last desperate attempt to get their attention. Nonetheless, no matter what he did, the churchgoers looked on unmoved, unimpressed, or even unconscious.

By the time his sermon was over, the church was half empty, and many of the parishioners who were left were sound asleep. Feeling totally defeated, the young pastor bowed his head and crept down from the pulpit a broken man. Just as he reached the bottom of the steps, an elderly woman who had been going to the church for years came up to him and said, "Young man, if you had gone up there like you came down, we would have listened to you."

God is BIG. There is no leader more farsighted, no boss more empowering, no book more motivating, no friend less judging, no family member more supporting, and no one who understands you more or knows your needs as well as God.

We, on the other hand, are quite small. We are extremely shortsighted in our thinking regarding our own lives and the lives of others. We are almost totally unaware of how our thoughts, actions, and interactions will impact the world and our future. If we depend on only what we see and understand, it will be impossible for us not to make error after error and confront failure after failure.

God is moving millions of people in billions of directions and knows the outcome of every move made. Humans have a God complex. We tend to fall into the trap of thinking that we are so brilliant, so judicious, and so capable that we can run the show for ourselves. However, we truly do not have even a glimmer of understanding of what God's will is in this world.

Until you change your viewpoint to "GOD, me" (BIG GOD, little me), you will often make it impossible for God's will to be done. Unless you can release all leadership responsibilities to God, you will stop His plan from achieving its ultimate success in your life, or in the lives of others. You will be creating stress instead of peace.

Do not rely on your own limited dimensions, or the limited dimensions of others. God is not only endlessly taller, He's endlessly longer, wider, and deeper. God is four-dimensionally unlimited. Rely on the unlimited God. Be *prideless* and realize what you see as the *right* way of thinking or acting may be totally or at least partially *wrong*. Try to look at things from God's perspective.

He is much BIGGER and can see much farther.

I've always been inspired by the fact that all the really cool, well-known athletes who came from the bottom and won championships and medals were people who always gave the glory to God. I also have always been inspired by the fact that all the really bad, well-known evil dictators who once were on top (but fell) always glorified *themselves*.

> God opposes the proud but gives grace to the humble. (James 4:6)

Where Credit Is Due

When my son, Skylar, was very young, I started trying to help him get some sense of God. Even at a very young age, he always had an amazing interest concerning spiritual matters. Unfortunately, what was more amazing was how much pride fit inside a three-year-old.

Each night before I put him to bed, I would ask some routine questions where I was looking for him to give God as an answer. One evening, to be funny, when I asked one of my typical questions, "Who made the moon?" he answered, "Skylar did it."

Then I said, "Come on, who made the moon?" Again he answered, "Skylar did it."

Next I said, "Then who made the sun?" To which he answered, "Skylar did it."

Finally, I said, "Come on, Skylar, who made the sun, the moon, and everything on the earth?" To which he answered once again, "Skylar did it."

The next evening, when I came home from my clinic and walked into the living room, I kicked over a sippy cup that was left on the floor and sent its contents flying all over the rug and wall. I immediately turned to Skylar and said, "Who left that cup on the floor?" To which he promptly answered, "God did it."

Needless to say, he got his first lesson in being *prideless* that night.

Philip Thinking vs. Andrew Thinking (or Man-Thinking vs. God-Thinking)

"When Jesus looked up and saw a great crowd coming toward him, he said to Philip [and Andrew], 'Where shall we buy bread for these people to eat?' He asked this only to test him [them], for he already had in mind what he was going to do" (John 6:5–6).

There are two ways Philip and Andrew could have looked at this question:

1. Man-Thinking
2. God-Thinking

Philip chose man-thinking and said, "Eight months' wages would not buy enough bread for each one to have a bite!" (6:7).

In other words, Philip was thinking, *Where will we find it? How can we afford it? What will we even feed them? What if we cannot handle this many people? But there isn't a McDonald's for miles . . . Where, how, what, what if,* and *but* are all man-thinking words and phrases. Man-thinking will always create excuses based on what appear to be limitations due to physical boundaries.

Andrew, on the other hand, chose God-thinking. He found a couple of pieces of Wonder Bread and some sardines and brought them to Jesus. While there was no way a man could have handled this problem, Jesus handled it easily—with food to spare.

God-thinking is not limited by time and space. God-thinking contains no excuses. God thinking knows, *"With God, all things are possible."*

> *Trust in the LORD with all your heart and lean not on your own understanding.*
> (Prov. 3:5)

INSTRUCTION #6: THOU SHALT BE TIMELESS

If You Think You're Always Running Out of Time, You Are Right

The goal of technology was to make work, travel, food preparation, and communication more time-efficient. This was done in an effort to give us *more* time. Regrettably that didn't seem to work out so well. Now, everyone feels as if they have *less* time.

You most likely wake up by an alarm, get paid by the hour, and eat by the clock. Everyone is always in a hurry. The dilemma is, this *feeling* that you have less time or are running out of time possibly creates more stress than any other one thing. The stress created by hurry is so intense, it can literally be deadly. *If you feel as if you are always running out of time, you're right.*

Owner's Manual Tip on Prideless Living: The Big Power of Prayer

Many of life's circumstances are so totally overwhelming that you cannot even begin to comprehend how you can change them. Often you will be too small to handle some of the world's BIG challenges. So don't. Turn them over to God. He is never too small, and no challenge is ever too great for Him to handle.

Turning things over to God is called *praying*.

After turning some *big* jobs over to God, eventually you may become so pleased with His work you'll end up turning *everything* over to Him.

You Feel Like You Are Always Running Out of Time If . . .

- *When you wake up* your mornings typically start out with instant oatmeal, microwaved waffles, and automatic coffee that brewed while you slept. Then you race off to work and get caught in rush-hour traffic. Because you can't wait to get to work to start making calls you use a cell phone. To save time, you use automatic speed dial.
- *When you are at work* you one-minute manage, make instant copies, have memos instead of meetings, use high-speed Internet access, and you page, beep, e-mail, or voice-mail people instead of waiting to actually talk to them. You take five-minute breaks, go out to lunch at restaurants that promise a ten-minute lunch, or order twenty-minute pizza delivery.
- *When you drive* you are constantly on the lookout for cops, get money from the automatic teller, and get pay-at-the-pump gas so you don't have to waste time going inside and actually interacting with someone.
- *When you come to a stoplight* you swerve into the lane with the least amount of cars. If there is a tie, you get behind what looks to be the latest model or fastest

car. If you can see the drivers, you get behind the youngest, most daring-looking one. Should someone hesitate at the green, he gets the wrath of your horn.

- *When you are hungry* you try to avoid shopping if you can by stopping at a convenience store or picking up some fast food.
- *When you get home at night* you watch news clips and instant replays of the life and the games you didn't have enough time to watch.
- *When you do have to go shopping* you try to get just enough food to go into the express lane. If this fails, you attempt to locate the smallest line. While in line, you watch people who got in a different line at the same time as you and pray that you beat them out of the store. Silently, you will the elderly lady in front of you to use cash instead of a check card and for the bagger to get a move on. If the lady fumbles around with her wallet or the bagger likes to talk, you begin to get stressed as you watch the people who got in the other lines at the same time as you begin moving ahead faster. If they beat you out of the store, you are actually a little depressed.

Today, the basic, underlying cause of stress would be anyone or anything getting in your way. Trying to defeat time has caused traffic, people cutting you off, the slow person in line, or any mode of transportation that is late to create not only stress, but potentially even *rage*.

Everyone is so busy. The problem is, if the beginning of your day is like someone just turned over an hourglass and you are trying to finish before the sand runs out, life is going to be stressful. Peace can come only when you realize that life is not a sprint; it's a marathon. Sprinting is hard, painful, and will not last very long. To finish the marathon of life you must go at a moderate, steady pace that can be kept up for a very long time and allows you to appreciate the landscape along the way.

If you think you are always running out of time, you are right. You cannot look at life as "short," or you will find yourself living a short life. Your time on earth is brief, but this should allow you to relax, not rush. Life is definitely not long enough to get that stressed over getting to the movies in time to catch the previews or arriving somewhere five minutes sooner than if you had actually driven the speed limit.

Our time on earth is temporary. Yet, it is also *complete*. In order to begin creating some peace in your life, you must begin to understand that God knows *what* you need and *when* you need it. By hurrying everything, you interfere with God's timing to try to meet your own schedule. As a result, you get "nowhere fast."

So slow down, take it easy, and try to enjoy the ride . . .

> You who say, "Today or tomorrow we will go to this or that city, spend a year there, carry on business and make money." Why, you do not even know what will happen tomorrow . . . Instead, you ought to say, "If it is the Lord's will, we will live and do this or that." (James 4:13–15)

The Hurry Illness

Instead of technology creating time, it has created illness, more specifically the *Hurry Illness*. With the dangers of stress we all face due to being in a hurry, the Hurry Illness is potentially a terminal disease.

In America, as people age, they do two things:

1. They move slower.
2. They move to Florida.

Because I live and practice in Florida, these two facts give me plenty of opportunities to test my quest to recover from the Hurry Illness. When I am rushing off to the office and get caught driving behind a slow-moving car being driven by a pair of elderly hands and no head, or if I am running through the airport and get behind someone in his nineties who is shuffling along, I attempt to recall that those situations are a lot like having God in front of me. He's older, wiser, and while He appears too slow at times, I always get there when I am supposed to. He never hurries, but He is always "right on time."

I consider myself to be a fairly capable human being. The problem, I have found, is that the things I make happen on my own never seem to bear the kind of fruit I had hoped for. My desire to help God, the world, my family, and myself frequently causes me to become impatient and want things to hurry along. When I am pushing things too fast, however, I usually find I have pushed myself right out ahead of God. When I do this, I end up making decisions that, in hindsight, I realize were either totally wrong or just not as good as they could have been. Also, because I am in front of God and not behind Him, I end up drawing all the fire and getting the most hurt.

God knows what He is doing. He is moving billions of people in billions of directions, trying to accomplish His will. When I am stuck, feeling rushed, frustrated, and noticing a case of the Hurry Illness coming on, I try to remember that "with the Lord a day is like a thousand years, and a thousand years are like a day" (2 Peter 3:8). Then I say to myself, "I am a patient man," and try to slow down long enough to let God take the lead.

When my Hurry Illness is in remission and I get and stay behind God, I usually manage to avoid a great deal of pain, failure, and suffering. Then, in His time, the right events, the right people, and the right decisions start coming into my life to make it successful again.

When you suffer from the Hurry Illness, you are simply rushing through your life. Soon the weeks become like days, and the years become like months. Pretty soon it is just New Year's to New Year's, with a whole lot of stress in between. The Hurry Illness causes you to microwave cook your life. Life goes fast, at extreme heat, and is done quickly. To save your life, stop, let God back in front of you, and remind yourself that, like Him, you are patient. This will add years to your life, and peace to your years.

It took the Israelites forty years to get across the desert, but they were behind God all the way. As a result, they got there right on *time*. I imagine God must have gotten awfully tired of hearing, "Are we there yet?"

The Present

Now there is nothing wrong. You cannot be upset about now. You can be stressed now, but it will be about results from the past or cares about the future. When you worry,

---

Owner's Manual Technology Alert

Cell phones, beepers, voice mail, and e-mail—oh my! We are electronically connected to everyone who knows us. Our electronic umbilical cords keep us fed with constant messages and requests that never allow our minds, or our time, to be free. It is the newest addiction. Like drugs, alcohol, sugar, or any other lethal addiction, it has the potential to ruin or shorten life.

The Time by God section of your *Owner's Manual* will show you how to manage your time, and when to turn your electronic umbilical cords on—and when to turn them off.

it's about before or later. Living for right now is God's gift of peace to you. That's why they call it "the present."

I once had a patient who, only in his midforties, had been told that due to his health condition, he could die at any moment. Every time he came in to see me he was understandably miserable. Then, one day, I noticed he'd had a tremendous change in attitude. Suddenly he was friendly, upbeat, and talkative. When I asked him what had caused this significant change of heart, he told me he'd realized that he had let a lot of good moments get past him worrying about what would happen next. Finally, he said that he had decided to focus on today and let "God take care of tomorrow."

Every time I saw him after that he would tell me, "It's been another good day." Soon, another good day turned into another good week and another good week turned into another good month and another good month turned into another good year.

Live in the eternal *now*. For in the eternal now, you have peace. *What a gift!*

> Therefore do not worry about tomorrow, for tomorrow will worry about itself. Each day has enough trouble of its own. (Matt. 6:34)

Don't Take the Game of Life Too Seriously

Your life is a game. Some people play the doctor game, some play the sales game, some play the athlete game, some play the student game, and some play the no job or ambition game. Some are kids, some are adults, some are married, some are single, some are parents, and some are a combination. But, no matter who you are or what you do, it is still a game.

Some games appear more important than other games. Surgeons have people's hearts in their hands, clergy have people's souls on their minds, and chiropractors watch their backs. A president's and a parent's work will determine the future, and a high-school dropout and a drug salesman may *have* no futures.

But it is still a game.

You can play the game to help move the world forward or backward. You can play the game to help create peace or chaos. You can give to the game or take from the game. But it is still a game.

You can appear to do better or worse in the game than others. You can get in great shape or out of shape, achieve or lose many things, create new ideas or never think at all, and become a pauper or a king. You can seem to beat others in many different ways or lose to others for many different reasons.

But it is still a game.

The reason your life is definitely a game is because, in the end, like any game, you go back in the box. No matter what type of game you played, how well you think you played it, what you won, who you lost to, or who you appeared to be, in the end, you go back in the box. Sooner or later, *time* is going to run out.

Eventually, you are going to die.

Usually, the goal of any game is to *win*. Nevertheless, the reality of life is that it is a game you can't really ever win. You can think you've won money, fame, houses, cars, hotels, Boardwalk, and Park Place, but in the end they become someone else's and you go back in the box. Knowing that, it really does not make sense to take yourself, or your time here, too seriously.

You should always play to win. Just remember that the real point of a game is not really annihilating your opponent, but to have as much fun as possible for as *long* as possible. If you're not having fun, you're not playing the game right—or you are not playing the right game. Don't waste time worrying about winning. The game moves pretty fast, so enjoy every moment of it you can. When the game of life is over, there are no overtimes or extra innings.

Make sure to play the game by the rules. Others deserve to enjoy the game and have a chance to win too. Since the game here doesn't last so long, you want to remember to think about what will happen when it's all over and you go back in the box.

Since you can't win and you can't lose, the only thing that makes sense is to risk everything, take every turn you can get, and always play your game full-out.

"Meaningless! Meaningless!" says the Teacher. "Utterly meaningless! Everything is meaningless." [It's just a game.] . . . So I commend the enjoyment of life, because nothing is better for a man under the sun than to eat and drink and be glad. Then joy will accompany him in his work all the days of the life God has given him under the sun. (Eccl. 1:2; 8:15)

Do not get too stressed if it's a long time between wins, or when you occasionally fall on your face. Just play the game at which you are best, the very best you can, and let the good times roll!

INSTRUCTION #7: THOU SHALT BE HATELESS

Forgiveness Is a Gift You Give Yourself

In Matthew, when Jesus healed the paralytic, He didn't smack him on the forehead and say, "Heal!" He said, *"You are forgiven."* That should clear up a lot of things for you. If you are forgiven, you are *healed.*

One of the most important things the Bible teaches us is that the first step to being forgiven is to become forgiving. It says not to bother praying, donating money, sacrificing your pets, or even getting out of bed unless you have forgiven everyone. That is explained in the statement: "For if you forgive men when they sin against you, your heavenly Father will also forgive you. But if you do not forgive men their sins, your Father will not forgive your sins" (Matt. 6:14–15).

Offering forgiveness is tough. Surely, it seems, there are certain acts and certain subhumans who are beyond or below forgiveness. Yet, at the same time, there must *not* be, because nowhere in the Bible is there a list of "unforgivable sins." If you have even one ex-friend, neighbor, or relative who you feel does not deserve forgiveness or one person who you feel is not above the wrath of your judgment, you cannot get well. Therefore, forgiveness is not just what you do for others; *"forgiveness is a gift you give yourself."*

In order to heal, you must remove all those shackles of judgment you have placed on everyone around you. Judgments like, *he's too big; she's too small; he's mean; she's so _____; he shouldn't _____; she's a bad _____; and those kids are _____* . . . all need to be eliminated.

If you do not unchain others from your judgment, neither will the chains of judgment be lifted from you. That's why it is also said, "Do not judge, or you too will be judged. For in the same way you judge others, you will be judged, and with the measure you use, it will be measured to you" (Matt. 7:1–2).

So, if you are judging with a bucket, you are being judged with a bucket, and if you are forgiving with a teaspoon, you are being forgiven with a teaspoon. In this case, you are definitely in harm's way. You will never heal, and your stress, your health, and your future don't stand a chance.

To get well, you must turn that around. Judge with a thimble and offer barrels full of forgiveness. Consequently, the same will be done unto you.

Judging and not forgiving may or may not cause harm to the recipients of those emotions, but the stress will certainly kill *you*. For that very reason, your peace and future lie in your own hands.

When you start forgiving and begin removing your judgment from others, you have begun to discover the greater part of loving and being *hateless*. This makes love no small task. But, despite the overwhelming challenges of loving, to love is not a suggestion; it's a command: "'Love the Lord your God with all your heart and with all your soul and with all your mind.' This is the first and greatest commandment. And the second is like it: 'Love your neighbor as yourself.' All the Law and the Prophets hang on these two commandments" (Matt. 22:37–40).

This Is My Command: Love Each Other (John 15:17)

It has always been assumed that you should "love your friends and hate your enemies." That seems pretty sound and simple. If you like me, I like you; if you don't like me or run over my cat, I hate you.

Regrettably, that's not what the Bible says—anywhere. It says, "Love your enemies and pray for those who persecute you" (Matt. 5:44).

Ouch, that's a tough one.

To put this into perspective, the "enemies" of whom Jesus was telling the Jewish people about in this part of the Bible were not just rude neighbors, telemarketers who call during dinner, kids who put gum on your seat, or people who annoy you at work. Jesus was speaking about the Romans. The Romans persecuted and abused the Hebrew nation in ways we could not even imagine today. They did this purely because the Jews believed in God and wanted to worship Him freely. The "enemies" Jesus told the people to love, and even pray for, were those who beat them, stole from them, imprisoned them unjustly, and murdered their children.

Loving the enemy or even just the incredibly annoying is where the rubber meets the road. Anyone can love the people who love them back. "Are not even the tax collectors [the liars, murderers, and thieves of society] doing that?" (Matt. 5:46). The love we are talking about here is God's love—the type of love that always forgives, limits judgment, and never ends. The type of love that heals you and will bring you peace.

"Love each other." Be hateless.

That's an executive order!

Love Each Vegetable?

Developing the capacity to be patient, tolerant, and compassionate toward even our worst enemies builds our ability to love. The most important part of expanding your ability to love is so that you also expand your ability to love God.

Love is an extremely difficult commitment. Love is constantly under fire. Your enemies, the people around you, and especially your family and friends will constantly challenge your ability to love them.

Most people would say that they are "loving." The problem is that their love has *limits*. God's love, the love He has commanded us to aspire to, is limitless and without condition. While you can upset Him and separate yourself from Him, He is slow to anger and quick to forgive. His love endures forever.

I was reminded of the limits and challenges involved with human love one evening when a family I was providing care for invited me over to dinner. When I arrived, both the adults were working hard in the kitchen and told me to have a seat in the living room. While I was sitting there looking at some books they had on the coffee table, their young daughter came running in to see me. She gave me a big hug and then said that her mother told her to ask me if I liked broccoli.

I said, "Broccoli? I love broccoli!"

The little girl responded, "I love broccoli too!"

For the next half hour, while dinner was cooking, she ran around the house, yelling and singing, "Broccoli, broccoli; I love broccoli."

When the meal was finally ready, I could barely wait to serve this girl some broccoli. Immediately after sitting down, I picked up the broccoli bowl and asked her how much she wanted. Her shocking reply was, "I don't want any."

Totally bewildered, I said, "You don't want any? I thought you loved broccoli."

To which she exclaimed, "I do love broccoli. But not enough to eat it."

Most of us love other people right up until we have to endure their issues and shortcomings. Then love ends, and judgment and unforgiveness begin. We love broccoli, but not enough to eat it.

"Love each other" is a tall order. People have their limits. Expect that. As you learn to love people despite their sometimes unlovable tastes, colors, or textures, you begin to love as God loves. He made broccoli and everything and everyone else on the planet—and He loves them all. God's love has no limitations, even though *people* often do. God wants you to get better at loving, because the better you get at loving others as He does, the better you also get at loving *Him*.

Loving is difficult, but it comes with a perk. As you learn how to get closer to people, you learn how to get closer to God.

To Love, Sometimes You Have to Get Down on Your Knees

Many of the people I have spoken with who have done charity work, gone on mission trips, or performed some kind of community service have told me that it did much more for them than it ever did for those in need. I have found this to be true in my own experiences as well.

I have had the opportunity to work with many charities over the years. The one that seemed to bless me the most was a small children's home. This place housed children from as young as age four or five all the way up to eighteen. The stories these kids told about their lives before coming to the home contained tragedies I never even imagined existed. Happily, to look at many of the kids, you would never know it. While some were bitter about their lives and resented their situation, others seemed totally content.

The reason so many kids got along well at the home was the loving environment the houseparents had created there. So powerful was the love of the people running the place that, eventually, even some of the most bitter children with the hardest pasts began to warm up.

One evening, all the kids were called down to the meeting hall. As the houseparents began to take roll call, they noticed that one of the boys from the younger group had not yet arrived. When they asked the other kids from his group where he was, they said he had crawled deep under one of the beds and would not come out.

Several of us went up there to see what was the matter with this boy. He happened to have a really challenging story and had not been fitting in well at the home at all. When we got to his room, we saw that he had wedged himself into the tiny little space underneath the bunk beds.

The first person to try to get him out was the lead parent from his group. She stood there and talked to the boy and lovingly tried to coax him out, but he would not move or even respond. After a few minutes, the gentleman who was the designated discipli-narian got frustrated. He stood there yelling at the boy and reminding him of the harsh punishment for those who do not listen or attend the meetings. Again, the boy did not move or respond.

We just stood there, baffled. Eventually, the head father from the home came in. He looked at us and looked at the situation and immediately dropped to his knees and crawled toward the bed under which the boy hid. He then pried his head under the bed and stuck out his hand. The little guy immediately grabbed the hand of the father and came out.

I learned some very important lessons that night. I learned that to truly love people, you have to get on their level. I also learned that sometimes, in order to love, you have to get down on your knees.

The Hateless Drill

Saying that you love people no matter who they are or what their circumstances are not a pious, holier-than-thou approach, in which you are thinking, *Because I am such a holy, godly person, I will love even the smallest, most ignorant of people.* It is not to say, "I love

---

The Hateless Drill

1. Make two columns.
2. In column 1, first write down all the really big things you hate or dislike about someone else.
3. Also in column 1, write down the little things humans do that upset you, like: leaving dirty underwear in the sink, wasting electricity, getting in the ten-item express-checkout line at the grocery store with twelve items, or parking in your flower bed.
4. In column 2, write down all the times you have done the same or similar things or made the same or similar mistakes listed in column 1.
5. Now that you see you are not better than the humans you are angry at or who cause you stress, but are actually the same, you can understand them, forgive them, stop judging them, and love them.

This exercise should be performed on a regular basis in order to maintain good health.

them because I am better than them." It is to say, "I love them because I am the same as them."

Think about it. What mistake, what sin, what stupid error in judgment have other people made that you have not made yourself? None. When I look at the people with whom I am angry, hateful, or unloving, I take note of the reasons behind those feelings. As a result, I always come to realize that, at some point in my life, I have done whatever it is I feel they have done to me.

When I get angry at someone cutting me off in traffic, I remember that I have done the same. If I am treated unkindly or unfairly, again, I remember when I have done the same. I have committed nearly every sin that has been committed against me at some point in my life. I am not better than anyone else, I am the same as them. When I realize that, I can act like the head father at the children's home or even the real head Father above. I can get on their level, hold out my hand, and love.

The Three Love Actions

Love is said to be the most powerful force in the world. It has been said that "God is Love." It has been said that "love conquers all." It has been said that "all you need is love." It has even been proved that without love, you cannot exist . . .

Love has been at the core of almost every poem, book, song, psalm, and movie since the beginning of time. Many authors, doctors, and researchers throughout history have dedicated their lives to searching for its source and its meaning.

In the Bible, love is described perfectly. Paul—the apostle, not the Beatle—said, "Love is patient, love is kind. It does not envy, it does not boast, it is not proud. It is not rude, it is not self-seeking, it is not easily angered, it keeps no record of wrongs. Love does not delight in evil but rejoices with the truth. It always protects, always trusts, always hopes, always perseveres. Love never fails" (1 Cor. 13:4–8).

Those verses can be heard at many weddings. Their description of love is very hard to beat, and it encompasses all the "10 Instructions for the Peace of God."

Looking deeper into the Bible, Moses and Jesus give us great examples of Paul's explanation of love in action. They showed us that to love you must do three things: *serve, sacrifice,* and *sustain.*

1. Serve. Moses served as the redeemer, leader, lawmaker, and prayer warrior of the entire Jewish nation. He personally saw to the safety and well-being of countless numbers of people and made sure they had food to eat, water to drink, and tents over their heads at night. Despite their constant complaining, negative attitudes, and continual lapses in faith, he dedicated himself to preserving their lives again and again—for four decades.

Jesus said He came to serve, not to *be* served. He showed us this by washing the feet of His disciples, who in those days had some pretty nasty feet. Back then, they wore only open-toed sandals and walked along dirt roads filled with garbage and refuse. It was considered common courtesy to wash the feet of visitors who came to your home. However, this job was typically reserved for the lowest-level servant in your employ. Jesus gave us the divine example of serving by scraping some pretty intense toe cheese off these people's feet. This included even Judas, a man who was to have Him crucified. (I don't think I am that loving. I can think of several things I would like to do to Judas's feet, and washing them is *not* one of them.)

2. Sacrifice. Moses left a life of Egyptian royalty to join a group of slaves. So deep was his love for his people, and for God, that he was willing to travel across a barren, scorching-hot desert for forty years at a time before bottled water, protein bars, drive-thrus, decent footwear, and port-a-potties.

Jesus sacrificed everything. Out of love, He endured public humiliation, torture, and an agonizing death.

3. Sustain. Moses had to sustain the people he loved through some pretty hot days, tired legs, confusion, and the fear of death. He let the Israelites know and kept them focused on the fact that on the other side of what appeared to be an endless desert was freedom and a land flowing with milk and honey. (These are just metaphors for prosperity, by the way. He did not mean dairy products and high-carbohydrate foods!)

Jesus had to sustain His followers through a desert of their own. The people who chose to follow Him were persecuted, beaten, stoned, jailed, and put to death. He encouraged them by promising not just a better life, but a better eternity. He promised them not only sugar and dairy products, He told them that on the other side of the desert was His Father's house, which contained mansions that already had mailboxes with their names on them.

Both Moses and Jesus served without condition *or* pay. They cast aside any pride by stepping down from any position of authority and subjecting themselves to public ridicule. They gave everything, up to and including their lives, to be shining examples of God's perfect love.

> *These three remain: faith, hope and love. But the greatest of these is love.* (1 Cor. 13:13)
>
> Sounds good to me . . .

INSTRUCTION #8: THOU SHALT BE FEARLESS

The Problems Ahead of You Are Never as Great as the Power Behind You

When God built the emotional sector of the mind into the BBG, He knew it would function in a world filled with challenge, change, and chaos. He never promised it would be easy, He promised only that He would be with you, every step of the way.

In order to believe you can overcome any obstacle, you must understand that *the problems ahead of you are never as great as the power behind you.*

BBG Owner's Tip: The Hold-Your-Tongue Rule

When attempting to live a life driven by love, you have to be constantly aware of your tongue during times of conflict. When you are in a disagreement with others, or someone makes a comment about you that you don't like or that hurts, it is time to follow the "Hold Your Tongue Rule." Saying something that hurts them back or tries to make you right never solves the conflict. It only makes sure that your relationship is damaged forever.

Live by the sword (tongue); die by the sword.

The tongue has the power of life and death. (Prov. 18:21)

God did not design the human mind to be weak and nonresistant to forces that occur outside it. Stress is not the enemy. Stress is dangerous only when you wrongly feel powerless against it.

Stress, no matter what the cause or reason, will not hurt you once you realize all the challenges and changes that occur in life can be not only survived, but overcome as well. The truth is, *only small-minded people are tamed by adversity; great minds rise above it.*

God does not allow a problem for which He has no solution. There is not a single crisis or circumstance that exists that someone has not triumphed over or gone around, and there is no disease that the body has not cured.

Life comes with built-in difficulties. *However, you can face life heroically, knowing God is behind you.*

> Be strong and courageous. Do not be terrified; do not be discouraged, for the LORD your God will be with you wherever you go. (Josh. 1:9)

It's "God's Life," Not Yours

Living life for God gives you freedom and fearlessness. When you turn your life and everything in it over to God, you have granted Him the opportunity and authority to bless it and take care of it in His way and His timing.

When things are not going smoothly with my work, my family, or my life in general, I say, "It's God's office," or, "God, this is Your family, life, etc." Then I have released it. If it's His, I can trust Him to handle the process as well as the results. All I have to do is show up and *fearlessly* do my job.

If things go poorly, I know it is God's will. When things go well and miracles happen, I say, "Praise God!"

He likes that.

When you take ownership over things in your life, you take control away from God. When He has no control, you do not allow His perfect will and plan to unfold in your life. You stop the blessings. So call your wife or husband, *"God's wife/husband,"* call your money, *"God's money,"* call your children, *"God's children,"* call your work, *"God's work,"* call your body, *"God's body,"* and call your life, *"God's life."*

When you turn everything over to Him, you glorify Him, and in God's time, the supernatural, right things will happen.

Again, He likes that.

> *The earth is the LORD's, and everything in it, the world, and all who live in it.*
> *(Ps. 24:1)*

Be Yourself, Only Better

When everything becomes God's and you have Him behind you, there is no enemy you cannot defeat and no task you cannot accomplish. Just look at David's "Three Mighty Men" (2 Sam. 23:8–12).

Mighty Man #1: Josheb-Basshebeth took up his spear against eight hundred men, whom he killed in one encounter.

Mighty Man #2: Eleazar took on the Philistines single-handedly as the other men of Israel retreated. He struck down Philistine after Philistine. When his hand grew tired, the Lord froze his hand to the sword. When the Israeli troops returned, all the Philistines were dead.

Mighty Man #3: Shammah and the Israeli troops were surrounded and vastly outnumbered by the Philistines. The Israeli troops fled, but Shammah stayed to defend God's territory, and he struck down the Philistines. The Lord gave a great victory that day.

When David was thirsty, the Three Mighty Men broke through the Philistine line to retrieve water and carry it back to David. David was so amazed by this miraculous feat and so taken by their loyalty and courage that he refused to drink the water.

Instead, "he poured it out before the LORD" (2 Sam. 23:16). *It's God's water.*

In addition to the Three, there were more than thirty mighty men of God in the Bible who won miraculous battles and accomplished great tasks through God. You become one of God's *fearless* Mighty Men when your life becomes "God's life."

Turn everything over to God and *be yourself, only better.*

> *I will protect him, for he acknowledges my name. He will call upon me, and I*
> *will answer him. (Ps. 91:14–15)*

The Five Steps to Fearlessness

When King Jehoshaphat (the son of David) found out that a vast, deadly, unbeatable army was about to destroy his country (a bigger problem than most of us typically have), he showed us the five steps to being fearless (2 Chron. 20).

Step 1: Take your problems to God. Some men came and told Jehoshaphat, "A vast army is coming against you from Edom, from the other side of the Sea.' . . . Alarmed, Jehoshaphat resolved to inquire of the LORD" (2 Chron. 20:2–3).

Step 2: Turn to God for answers to your problems. Jehoshaphat said, "O our God, will you not judge them? For we have no power to face this vast army that is attacking us. We do not know what to do, but our eyes are upon you" (2 Chron. 20:12).

Step 3: Remember that it's God's battle, not yours. The Lord said, "Listen, King Jehoshaphat and all who live in Judah and Jerusalem! This is what the LORD says to you: 'Do not be afraid or discouraged because of this vast army. For the battle is not yours, but God's'" (2 Chron. 20:15).

Step 4: With God be fearless (strong and courageous). The Lord continued, "Tomorrow march down against them. They will be climbing up by the Pass of Ziz, and you will find them at the end of the gorge in the Desert of Jeruel. You will not have to fight this battle. Take up your positions; stand firm and see the deliverance the LORD will give you, O Judah and Jerusalem. Do not be afraid; do not be discouraged. Go out to face them tomorrow, and the LORD will be with you" (2 Chron. 20:16–17).

Step 5: Let God be glorified in victory, and let the blessings flow. "When the men of Judah came to the place that overlooks the desert and looked toward the vast army, they saw only dead bodies lying on the ground . . . There was so much plunder that it took three days to collect it. On the fourth day they assembled in the Valley of Beracah [*Beracah* means "praise"], where they praised the LORD . . . And the kingdom of Jehoshaphat was at peace, for his God had given him rest on every side" (2 Chron. 20:24–26, 30).

INSTRUCTION #9: THOU SHALT BE FAITHFUL

It's Not What You Know, It's Who You Know

You cannot have Peace by God if you do not even *know* God is there. To have strong peace, you've got to have strong faith.

There Are 3 Types of Faith:

1. **"I Will Believe It When I See It" Faith.** If you need to see God or have a need for God to perform magic, signs, or miracles to believe in Him, then you have *no faith*.

2. "Believer" Faith. You can believe only what you do not see. If you merely believe, then you have *weak faith.*

3. "Ph.D." (Past Having Doubt) Faith. When you have Ph.D. faith, you are Past Having Doubt. When you *know* God is as real as the chair you are sitting in, the bed you are lying in, or the floor you are standing on, and you see concrete evidence of Him in all things, you have *strong faith.*

The Bible describes faith as "the substance of things hoped for, the evidence of things not seen" (Heb. 11:1 NKJV). In order to have strong faith, you must start *knowing* that God will provide for your needs and answer your prayers. You must literally, physically see the substance of your hopes and dreams as if they are right there in front of you.

Faith that must be seen is not faith. *Just as you don't need to see air in order to breathe, you don't need to see God in order to have faith.* Needing evidence for faith is *not* faith. Even when there are no miracles or magic tricks, God is still *there.*

If you are an "I will believe it when I see it" person or a "believer" person, you have faith that relies on sight and faith that relies on faith. Neither of these is really faith at all. *The faith that relies on God is the only faith there is.*

To work on your Ph.D. in God, there are some things you can do:

- When you are outside, think about the "out of this world" power and splendor of nature. Some people look at a tree and see how much lumber they could get and sell from it, some see it as pretty, some see it as in the way, and some do not even take the time to see it at all. When you start to look at the tree in awe and see it as evidence of God's incredible power, wisdom, and ability, you are beginning to see God and His presence in this world.
- Consider the tremendous organization of our bodies and the universe we live in. Consider the kidney. Contemplate the fact that the kidney possesses many different kinds of cells and that each cell was designed for different kinds of functions. Each of these functions plays a different role in the overall health of the kidney, and the overall life of literally the entire body. With that kind of organization, there has to be an Organizer. There has to be a God.
- Talk to God as you would talk to someone who is really there. Because He is.

Practice these three things every day in order to become more *faithful*. While few of us, if any, will ever graduate with a Ph.D., as you get to *know* God better, you will begin to graduate from experiencing an enormous amount of fearful stress.

> By faith we understand that the universe was formed at God's command, so that what is seen was not made out of what was visible. (Heb. 11:3)

The Manna Principle: Exercise Your Faith

Challenges present the greatest opportunities to build faith. When you are challenged and you turn to God for answers and deliverance rather than fearing and complaining, you build your faith. Challenges are "faith exercises."

When Moses was called by God to move the Israelites out of the bonds of slavery, he was faced with many challenges. Of course, the most significant of these challenges was the lack of food. People get cranky when they are hungry.

When the people in the desert began to be confronted with the challenge of potential starvation, rather than showing faith by turning to God, they did the opposite. They became miserable, whined, and feared the worst.

Moses, on the other hand, exercised his faith. When he was faced with the challenge, he *did* go to God. As a result, God blessed Moses and the Israelites by providing bread from heaven called "manna."

Although God provided food, He still called for faith. He allowed the people to collect only enough manna for one day. If they collected more, the additional food rotted. In this way, they had to renew their faith in the Lord every day.

Each day, they had to *exercise their faith*.

Following the "Manna Principle" means turning to God in times of stress and having faith that He will answer your prayers one day, one problem, or even one *meal* at a time.

> If you do not stand firm in your faith, you will not stand at all. (Isa. 7:9)

What Is Your "Brix" Reading?

In an effort to grow better, tastier produce, fruit and vegetable growers use different ways of measuring quality. One barometer of testing that can be used on fruits and vegetables is called a refractometer. When you place some liquid from a particular piece of produce into the refractometer, it measures the concentration of sugar in the liquid. The measurement you get is called a "Brix" reading. The higher the "Brix" reading, the higher the quality of the produce, and the juicer and tastier it will be.

When testing *people* for quality, just like produce, the best way to test them is by "squeezing" them. Like a vegetable or a piece of fruit, people may appear to look good on the outside, but it is quite another thing once you open them up.

It is easy to be peaceful, kind, helpful, and loving when things are status quo, but it is quite another to be that way when you are *squeezed*. The true test of what is inside you is not what you are like when things are going your way, it is what you are like when you are awakened at four in the morning, when you wreck your car, when you lose your keys, or when you stub your little toe. Those are the types of moments that truly reveal who you are. It is during the tough times that you are put under the God refractometer and your "Brix" reading is revealed.

The God refractometer does not check your tastiness or juiciness; it tests the quality and the quantity of your commitment to Him. The higher the "Brix," the higher the concentration of God in you, and the more "fruitful" your life will be.

When you squeeze an orange or an apple, no matter the time or situation, orange juice and apple juice come out. I have never squeezed an orange and gotten milk. Sadly, often throughout my life when *I've* been squeezed, rather than God coming out, out came something entirely different.

To change my low "Brix" readings, I have tried to commit every large and small area of my life to God. When I wake up, I say good morning to God. Before I eat, I dedicate the meal to God and ask Him to bless it. I pray before everything and *for* everything. My only true priorities are the things in my life that truly bless and serve Him. Everything else is just a hobby.

Over time, my increased focus on my commitments to God has caused me to become more filled with God and develop higher "Brix" readings. Now, when I am cut off at an intersection, spill food on my shirt, get treated rudely by a waitress, or have a problem in a relationship, I am more likely to have God come out and less likely to have the ugly, horrifying, three-eyed stress monster come out.

While I know I will never reach it, I am always striving for a 100-percent "Brix" reading—the most peaceful, tasty, *juicy* life possible.

Make a tree good and its fruit will be good, or make a tree bad and its fruit will be bad, for a tree is recognized by its fruit . . . For out of the overflow of the heart the mouth speaks. The good man brings good things out of the good stored up in him, and the evil man brings evil things out of the evil stored up in him. (Matt. 12:33–35)

Are You a Rhino, a Boar, or a Llama?

The Rhino: The rhino has massive girth, blazing speed, and extremely dangerous weaponry. If the rhino is attacked or threatened, it charges.

The Boar: The boar is only about four feet long and three feet high; however, its lower teeth grow into tusks that, while mostly designed for digging, can present a significant danger to humans or other animals. If the boar is attacked or threatened, it also charges.

The Llama: The llama has a relatively small stature and contains no battle skills, weaponry, or defense systems of any kind. The llama has no real power or ability. Despite all that, when an enemy threatens, just like the boar and the rhino, the llama charges.

Because of its incredible power, the rhino has full faith in itself. This is *no faith*. Despite its abilities, a skilled hunter can always bring down the rhino; therefore, the rhino now faces extinction.

Regardless of its limitations, the boar charges because it still has faith in its own weapons. This is *weak faith*. Despite its abilities, most any hunter will defeat the boar, and as a result, the boar population has become limited in certain parts of the world.

The llama has absolutely no power, and thus could not possibly have any faith in its own ability to fight. Even though the llama has absolutely no game, he knows "God's got game." This animal charges enemies it could not possibly defeat, totally relying on God that this tactic will win. The llama has *strong faith*. Predators see the confidence with which the llama charges and retreat!

As a result of its faith, the llama is alive in abundance today.

Superman is not courageous. He has no fear. He is the man of steel and he knows he cannot be hurt. Courage doesn't mean you are not afraid. It means you *are* afraid—and you do what you have to anyway. Courage means that while you know you are weak, you know you can be hurt, and you know you don't have much game, you charge straight ahead anyway. You do this because you have faith that God is strong and will bring you victory.

It's not faith if you know you can do it! Don't be a rhino or a boar; be a llama. With llamalike faith, you can charge head-on into your life.

When you are *faithful*, you are the true Superhero.

Faith is courage under fire . . .

INSTRUCTION #10: THOU SHALT BE HOPEFUL

Hope to Win

The only reason a sheep tender named David dared to face the giant Goliath was because he was *hopeful*. When the giant laughed at David and told him he would feed his intestines to the birds, because David had *hope*, he laughed right back and told him he would feed *his* intestines to the birds. Because he had *hope*, David even went so far as to take off his armor, throw down his sword, and take on the fiercest of all enemies with nothing more than a *rock*.

With Hope, You Are Daring

Rather than making excuses for why it would be impossible or even dangerous for you to overcome the stress in your life, with hope, you can be daring enough to make whatever moves are necessary to get past your obstacles.

With Hope, You Are a Dreamer

Whatever you feel is possible *is* possible. Whatever you think is impossible *is* impossible. With hope, you never shoot anywhere but high, and you never think any way but *big*.

Owner's Manual Tip for Hope

Nothing is more certain than this: *the defeat of someone who quits . . . and the victory of someone who never will.*

With Hope, You Are Courageous

Success usually comes with a heavy price tag. It costs time, it costs money, and it may even cost some relationships. However, if it serves God, serves you, and serves the world, then it is worth it. Whatever you do, it will take courage. Whatever path you take, if it is a winning path, there will always be someone to tell you that you are wrong. With hope, do it anyway.

With Hope, You Are Different

Always remember that the *popular* path is usually the *wrong* path. God's path will usually lead you a *different* way, but only God's path leads the *right* way. Do not let the hopeless lead you astray.

With Hope, It's Okay to Fail

If everything is going *your* way . . . you are probably going the *wrong* way. On the road to a better life, you *will* get knocked down. With hope, you know that God will be there to pick you up again and again.

If You Hope, You Win . . .

"But those who hope in the LORD will renew their strength. They will soar on wings like eagles; they will run and not grow weary, they will walk and not be faint" (Isa. 40:31).

If Life Keeps Throwing You Curveballs, Learn to Hit Curveballs

When I played in the thirteen-year-old division in Little League baseball, life was good. I was one of the best players in the league and chosen to be on the All-Star Team. During that season, if someone threw a pitch over the plate, I could hit it anytime and to almost anywhere I wanted.

I went into the next season ready to make my mark among the fourteen-year-olds. I stepped up to the plate for the first time that year with confidence. I was ready to pounce on the first pitch and try to knock it right out of the park. Much to my dismay, the pitcher threw the first ball right at my head. However, just as I was ducking away and thinking that it was a lousy pitch, the ball took a sharp right turn and crossed directly over the plate for a strike.

It turned out that the pitchers in the fourteen-year-old division threw curveballs!

Things suddenly became very stressful for me. Life had literally thrown me a curveball. Any pitcher who could throw a curveball could strike me out. Each time I struck out, I would storm back to the dugout and blame curveballs for my misfortune. I did this again and again until one day, my coach came over to me and said, "Ben, the problem is not the curveball. The problem is that you cannot hit the curveball."

It then occurred to me that other people could hit that pitch. Suddenly, I had hope. The coach then showed me how to hit this difficult pitch. He taught me that the key to hitting a curveball was to move up in the batter's box toward the pitch and hit it before it curved.

Hitting curveballs is just like life. First you have hope. You realize that other people have had the same or even worse challenges than you and have been able to overcome them. Then you stop ducking away or sitting back and waiting for problems to defeat you. Instead, you step up to the problems, and hit them before they hit you.

P.S. I never could hit curveballs that well, and I did continue to strike out sometimes. But I made the All-Star Team again that year anyway. Because, just like life, baseball isn't all curveballs; you can strike out once in a while and still be an All-Star.

> *Let us not become weary in doing good, for at the proper time we will reap a harvest if we do not give up [stay hopeful]. (Gal. 6:9)*

Turn: Your Oppositions into Opportunity, Your Fears into Fascination, and Your Errors into Education

Maintaining a *hopeful* attitude is one of the greatest determining factors of your health, relationships, success, and peace of mind. On your quest for treasure, very often you will get rocks. Nevertheless, it is up to you whether or not those rocks are immovable obstacles or stepping-stones.

I like to get to my clinic about half an hour before it opens so I can get settled in and focus my mind on the tasks of the day and the needs of my patients. Because it is so early, it is usually still dark when I leave my house. One morning I got in my truck and starting it, I noticed that it still seemed awfully dark inside the vehicle. Confused, I played around with the overhead lights, the headlights, and even tried starting the truck over again to see if that would solve the problem. Then it struck me: All the lights were out on the dash where the radio was.

Or should I say, had been . . .

When I reached down to find out why the radio lights were off I discovered it was because my radio was gone! Someone had broken into my vehicle overnight and ripped the radio right out of my car and stolen all my tapes and CDs.

Just as I was about to begin the freaking-out process, I realized that I had a decision to make. I could let this ruin my entire morning, day, or even week, or I could not. I decided not to. I said to myself, "This will give me an opportunity to drive to the office in silence and spend some extra time in prayer."

I turned opposition into opportunity.

Meanwhile, the original radio was replaced with an even better one by my insurance company about a week later.

Fearful times can become fascinating when you see them as puzzles to be solved and a chance to test your faith. I have always spent a good part of my time traveling around the world speaking. Before the events of 9/11, which significantly changed air travel, I had gotten pretty good at the art of airport timing. I knew exactly when to leave my home or office so I could get to my gate precisely on time.

On my first trip after the 9/11 disaster, I got to the airport exactly when I usually do. The problem occurred when I discovered that the line at security was huge. It literally wrapped around the terminal—twice. Rather than fearing that I would miss my flight, throw off my schedule, and possibly not reach my destination, I thought, *My plane leaves in thirty minutes, and I'm in a ninety-minute line. I am now fascinated.* I decided to turn the experience into a faith tester. It was a fascinating chance to see if God wanted me home—or at a seminar.

After only ten minutes in line, someone from the airline brought all those who had flights leaving soon to the front, and I made it to my gate right on time.

Early on in my career, I impatiently invested in a business opportunity before all the facts were in. As a result, I lost more money than I thought was even possible to lose.

For a while, I was devastated by the error I had made and what it had cost me. I beat myself up for over a year until I finally saw what I had learned through the entire ordeal that I could put toward my future. I started to look at it as an education instead of an error. Of course, for what I spent, I could have gone to Harvard graduate school thirty times over, but I know that I will easily make that back because of what I learned from the experience.

Seeing the world as fearful, depressing, and full of opposition and failure doesn't solve anything. Amazing discoveries are always precluded by trial, research, and investigation.

So stay *hopeful*.

Worry about nothing; pray about everything . . .

Affirmation: It's Hope Through God, Not Just a Positive Mental Attitude

Sometimes things just do not work out. Having a "Positive Mental Attitude" (PMA) usually means you are figuring everything will eventually go your way. Regrettably, sometimes it won't. PMA is Peace by Man, not Peace by God.

Being *hopeful* is more than just being positive. Being hopeful means no matter what happens, you trust God has a plan that will *always* work for the ultimate good—even when you have no idea what God is doing with your life or if He is even a part of your life. It may not be *your* plan, but it *will* be the best plan for you—and everyone around you. Therefore, you have hope no matter what the situation appears to be or what type of circumstance you are in.

In order to live in this world, you will have to overcome monstrous injustice and fierce opposition. On the other hand, God loves you. He loves you even more than *you* love yourself. You will be tested, and it will most likely not occur when or how you wanted. But, when you know that God loves you and He deeply desires that your life work out, you have hope. Come what may.

When a child is taking drugs, failing school, or headed in the wrong direction, the father of that child loves that child's body, life, and future more than the child does. It is exactly the same with your Father-God. When He sees you in trouble or falling short of your potential, He wants much more for you than even *you* do. That is why the Bible says, "The LORD your God is with you; the mighty One will save you. He will rejoice over you. You will rest in his love; he will sing and be joyful about you" (Zeph. 3:17 NCV). It says He not only loves you, He rejoices and is joyful about you. He even sings about you. It is very unlikely that you love yourself so much that you are willing to sing about yourself.

But God *does* love you that much.

No matter how steep or treacherous it gets, keep moving up the mountain with your eyes focused on God. Keep moving up the mountain with your family, your health, your relationships, your finances, and your dreams. When you are stressed because you're running late, worried that you may run out of money, or something is going wrong with your family, job, or your life, be hopeful. God wants you to get to the top even more than *you* do.

It is through your eyes, your mouth, and your hands that God often gets things done in this world. If you become anxious and lose hope, His will cannot be done. A lot of people say this affirmation: "I can do this with God's help."

Then again, often the *right* affirmation is, *"With my help, God can do this."*

> I have learned to be content whatever the circumstances [hope defined]. (Phil. 4:11)

THE BODY BY GOD 40-DAY PLAN FOR MANAGING STRESS (CREATING PEACE)

Stressors come and stressors go. There's nothing you can do about traffic jams, inclement weather, job layoffs, rude employees, or your favorite football team's losing

Owner's Manual Guide to Implementing the 10 Instructions and Managing Stress

The Time Management section in your *Owner's Manual* will show you when and how to make time for spiritual growth and perception upgrades. During those times, make sure you read some or all of "The 10 Instructions for Peace by God." As you read the instructions over and over again, you will begin to understand them more, and they will become more deeply engrained in your mind and your emotions. In time, the result will be more peace.

Time by God: "The Time Zones" contains strategies for putting certain actions into place that will help you to have fewer stressful circumstances. This will allow you not only to manage your stress, but to shrink and contain it.

score on Sunday afternoon. But what you *can* change is how you react to those stressors that, once upon a time, worked as triggers for your BBG's negative stress reactions.

See the Body by God 40-Day Plan in the Life by God section to begin creating peace and seeing your stress improve 1 percent each day for forty days. Anyone can get 1 percent better a day at relating to people, relaxing in times of chaos, and seeing the world from a better point of view.

When it comes to seeing the world from a higher vantage point, seeing your life from the top of the mountain down, and looking back from the head of the class, it will take time. There are no quick fixes to stress management. There are no "overnight successes" when it comes to creating peace.

PART FIVE | TIME MANAGEMENT FOR YOUR BODY BY GOD

19 | TIME BY AND FOR GOD

The Key to Reducing Stress, Creating Health, and Building a Life by God

Managing your time is perhaps the most significant aspect of managing your life. If you had forty-eight hours a day to get things done instead of twenty-four, your stress would already be reduced, you'd eat less fast food, and you'd probably even exercise more. Although it may not appear that way right now, this is possible. The time is there; all you have to do is get twice as much use out of your time.

Much of your time is centered around handling all the issues and "emergencies" you face with your relationships, your health, your work, and your stressful outlook on life. In a life like that, you end up so focused on just getting *through your day* that you forget about getting *from your day*. The result of that kind of focus is more issues and "emergencies" that use up even more time.

The following Time Management chapters will show you how to organize and strategize your time so it is focused on activities that build a healthy, happy, peaceful, and successful life—a "Life by God." This is the key to stress management, relationship building, financial increase, appearance enhancement, and health control. By continuously working to create a Life by God, you reduce the amount of stress that keeps popping up in your world and develop a Body by God that doesn't get sick, tired, or out of shape. You will learn in this part of the manual how to begin working *on* your life, instead of working in your life on all of your issues and emergencies. Over time, this will create less and smaller issues and emergencies, allowing you to continue focusing more of your time on what you are passionate about and what and who is important.

ARE YOU MANAGING YOUR TIME?
OR IS YOUR TIME MANAGING YOU?

Time by Man or Time by God?

Typically, *you are not managing your time; it is managing you.* In fact, the constant crises and deadlines of your thoroughly modern day are most likely determining your each and every move—and managing your time, your body, and your emotions.

When you woke up this morning, it is likely that the very first things you thought of were not those things necessary to create time for exercise, better nutrition, and peace by God. Instead, from the moment you opened your eyes, you were probably thinking of those things that were so vital they had to be handled *immediately.* As time went on, you most likely spent the rest of your day handling urgent issues, meeting deadlines, managing relationship breakdowns, and attempting to get to places *on time.*

Most people would consider this "effective" time management. They have organized their day so the most important and pressing issues are being handled first, and so they are not late to anything.

However, this is not really "time management," it is "emergency management." In emergency management, your *time* manages *you.* When your time is managing you, that is Time by Man. Time by Man leaves precious little time for what is *really* important in life, which is Time by God. Time by Man causes you to just get through the day while Time by God allows you to get from the day.

Time by God is managing your time so you can do what is necessary to create health, peace, success, better relationships, or anything else that is good for your future.

To begin following some of the rules, directions, and guidelines in your *Owner's Manual for Maximized Living,* you must learn to manage your time so you have enough time for getting your life back under control.

THE "TIME ZONES"
HOW TO GET 160 HOURS FROM A 40-HOUR WORKWEEK

ZONE 1
TIME BY MAN

• EMERGENCY CENTERED (TIME, RELATIONSHIPS, PERSONAL)
• SURVIVAL DRIVEN • REACTIVE FOCUSED

DISTRACTIONS: Technology and Hobbies, News and World events, Treatment for Illness, Emotional Challenges, Fringe Business

ZONE 2
TIME BY GOD

• MISSION CENTERED • PRINCIPLE DRIVEN
• CAUSE-ACTIVE FOCUSED

MISSION-ARY WORK: Healthy Lifestyle, Spiritual Growth, Relationship Building, Social and Community Involvement, Skill Sharpening and New Skill Development, Opportunity, Planning & Organizing, Coaching, Maintenance, Perception Reprogramming

To Have Time for My Four Full-Time Jobs, I Must Find Time by God

I take care of patients, I write, I am a speaker/consultant, and I am also focused on maintaining a thriving family and athletic life. I really have four full-time jobs. To do all the things I do *full-time*, I need to get 160 hours out of a 40-hour work-week. While I am able to take good care of my patients, have a quality family life, successful business ventures, and stay in top, competitive shape, most people I work with don't feel they have the time to do even *one* thing with excellence. The truth is that all people have the time; they just don't know how to *manage* the time effectively.

The Time by God system will show you how to get in and stay in great health, be a successful student, focus on career, and be an incredible spouse and parent, without feeling that you are using more time than you are right now. To get four times more done in a week than you ever thought possible, you must begin using time the way God intended. You must begin *using* Time by God and stop *spending* Time by Man.

"With the Lord a day is like a thousand years, and a thousand years are like a day" (2 Peter 3:8). Time by God may not get you 1,000 hours out of a day, but, like me, it *will* start to help you get 160 hours out of a 40-hour week.

ZONE 1: TIME BY MAN

Zone 1 is centered on handling time, relationships, and personal emergencies. Behavior in this zone is driven by the desire to meet the basic needs of survival in the most pleasing, easiest way possible.

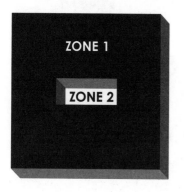

The focus in Zone 1 is placed on *reacting* to these emergencies and distractions or whatever else is necessary to meet these survival needs.

This is the "Time by Man" zone. The energy spent in Zone 1 is used to satisfy man's worldly physical, material, and emotional wants and curiosities.

In the diagram on the previous page, the arrows of Zone 1 point "in" because the more time you spend handling the emergencies of "Time by Man," the less time is left over for "Time by God." The larger Zone 1 gets, the smaller Zone 2 gets.

Living in Zone 1

Due to the survival mode built in to us, the goal of humankind tends instinctually to be to put the best food on the table, the sweetest shoes on our feet, the most stylish clothes on our back, and the nicest roof over our heads in the cheapest, easiest, quickest way possible. Our primitive wants are for less work for more pay, fast food, immediate service, a quick buck, instant coffee, and instant relief. If possible, people would like all this without ever getting off the couch. Often there are those who want these things so badly, they are willing to put aside any morals, principles, or sensitivity to others to get them.

The success of fast-cash home businesses, illegal and legal drugs, fast-food chains, convenience stores, pizza delivery, Internet shopping, bars, and casinos, and the resultant failure of our financial security, health, fitness, families, and peace of mind are all based on this natural, instinctive survival mode. This is all Zone 1 living.

Our basic human tendency is to deviate into Zone 1, Time by Man. When I am working with the sick, the overweight, and/or the depressed, I always find that in some way, on some level, they are stuck in a mode of getting things as easily, as quickly, and as satisfyingly as possible. In many instances, this is done without any real focus on ethics, the lives of others, God, or the future. It is usually quite clear to me that their most considerable crisis is due to this Zone 1 living.

A great example of this type of living exists in many of us when we are in one of our most primitive states, as seniors in high school. The typical high-school senior cannot wait to finally leave the home, flee from the boundaries set by his or her parents, and get life started. The problem is, many want to get life started the easiest, quickest way possible and skip some of the tougher steps in between—like going to college, finishing with a degree or degrees, and/or gaining some experience in the real financial world.

I must know dozens of people who after high school wanted to avoid the work of continuing their education. They were in such a hurry to get out, start a family, and begin making some money that they took what they thought was the easy way out. They ended up very quickly taking jobs they were not passionate about but made them what appeared to be good money and created for them what seemed to be an easy life at the time.

I have many friends and patients who are now married with several children and have found that the jobs and opportunities they got right out of high school may have seemed good then, but now no longer meet their mental, emotional, or financial needs. They struggle to get by, are miserable at work, and have a tremendous amount of stress and tension in their home lives that seem inescapable.

These people are loved by God and still, to this day, have hope and a future. Unfortunately, some have just shrunken down and accepted their fate. While others I know have attempted to seek solutions, the problem is that they seek them in the wrong places. They try to solve the troubles they created through having a Zone 1 life with more of Zone 1 living. They look for ways out by trying to make a quick buck, trying to just make life easier somehow, quitting their jobs, quitting their families, or just simply fleeing from their responsibilities. None of these steps ever help anyone find a better life, because you cannot solve a crisis by living the same way you were living when the crisis was created.

What is needed is to flee Zone 1 living and begin Zone 2 living.

ZONE 2: TIME BY GOD

Time spent in Zone 2 is centered on discovering and working on your mission. *Your mission is how you will develop and use your God-given gifts to serve God in making this a better world.*

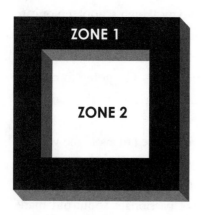

Behavior in this zone is driven by principles and a commitment to the moral and ethical code of the mission.

The focus of Zone 2 is cause-active. The activities of the day are initiated and fueled by a personal desire to create change in your life, improve the lives of others, and manage your world in a way that causes success and prevents crisis.

Zone 2 is the "Time by God" zone. The cares and concerns of Zone 2 are spiritual and eternal; not material and temporary. God's time involves your own change, growth, and well-being, as well as that of others.

In the diagram on page 291, the arrows of Zone 2 point "out" because the more "Time by God" you spend, the less emergencies there are, and the less "Time by Man" you will need to spend. The larger Zone 2 becomes, the smaller Zone 1 becomes.

Moving to Zone 2, the Right Time Zone

If you moved to a new time zone and never changed your watch *or* your schedule, you would always be early or late, forever eating breakfast while other people were eating lunch or dinner, and consistently missing your bus. Your life would continually be "off."

If you are living in Zone 1, Time by Man, no matter how much you try to improve, succeed, or manage your stress, you will still always be "off." That is because Zone 1 is simply the *wrong* Time Zone.

The more time you spend in one zone, the less time you have left for the other. If you are focusing your life on reacting to the emergencies of Zone 1, you shrink the time you have to spend cause-actively preventing them in Zone 2. Ironically, the more time you spend reacting to trouble, the more trouble you end up having.

When emergencies control your time, your time controls you.

Effectively pursuing a better life results from spending the largest amount of time in Zone 2, the Time by God zone. This is the *right* Time Zone for developing the areas that help to improve who you are, and assist you in your health, fitness, relationships, and financial future. All this allows you to better the world.

Obviously, the ideal way of life would be to have always lived in Zone 2 so you do not end up in the situation created by Zone 1 living where you have a job you dislike, a family that is struggling, severe financial limitations, and all kinds of emotional and health concerns. The encouraging news is, however, Zone 1 is never truly inescapable. By beginning to force some of your life into Zone 2, you begin to eliminate many of the emergencies of Zone 1. Things like going back to school, starting to work out, eating Food by God, and reading the 10 Instructions for Peace by God will start to shrink Zone 1 and expand Zone 2.

God always gives you a way out without having to flee from your responsibilities. As a matter of fact, it is when you confront the responsibilities that you were avoiding because of your tendency to live in the Time by Man zone instead of the Time by God zone, that life begins to change for the better. You begin to shrink your problems and swell your solutions.

The Cradle Paradox

When I was in eighth grade, I joined my junior high school wrestling team. From the moment I stepped onto the mat for the very first time, I fell in love with the sport. While at first glance it may appear to be a game where two people in tights roll around and sweat all over each other, the reality is that wrestling is potentially the most complex, physically demanding sport that exists. There are literally hundreds of offensive and defensive moves involved in wrestling, with countermoves designed to stop each one of them.

There are also counters to each of those counters . . .

The objective in wrestling is to try to catch someone in one of your moves more often then he catches you in one of his moves. If you get caught, you then need to figure out a counter move so you can get out. Unfortunately, as a beginning wrestler I spent most of my time working on my counter moves.

In my third match of that very long and painful eighth-grade season, I got caught in a very difficult move called a "cradle." The cradle happens when your opponent puts you on your back by pulling your knee up against your nose and locking his arms around your head and your leg. No matter how hard I tried, kicked, or screamed, I could not get out of it. Eventually, my opponent pinned my back to the mat, and the match was over.

Afterward, I asked my coach how to get out of (counter) a cradle. He said, "Easy. Don't end up in one in the first place."

BBG Owner's Warning

Like many problems and stressors in life, the problem with a cradle is that it is a sneaky move. You can be about to be placed in a cradle and not even know it. Therefore, always do your best to keep your nose away from your knee (spend Time by God in Zone 2). *Trust me on this one.*

If I had done what I was supposed to do as a wrestler and built a solid foundation by being in the right position, doing the right training, working hard enough in practice, learning and developing the right skills, and keeping my nose away from my knee, I would have never ended up in a cradle and been pinned in the first place.

Most people look at emergencies the way I used to look at wrestling in the eighth grade—by thinking, *How do I get out of trouble?* The reality is, most problems and emergencies are just like getting locked in a cradle: The best cure is not to end up in them in the first place! If you do, chances are you are going to get pinned.

Do what you are supposed to do by building a solid foundation for your life through centering your time on Zone 2, Time by God. That way, you do not end up always trying to figure out ways of countering the emergencies of Zone 1, Time by Man.

If you do not think you can ever get out of the predicaments you are in, note that I did later learn there are some things you can do to get out of a cradle. They are really difficult to do; they are uncomfortable, and often involve biting and scratching, but it can be done. There is always a way out.

TIME BY MAN VS. TIME BY GOD: "BE IN THE WORLD, NOT OF IT . . ."

You have a choice of two BBG Time Zones in which to focus your time and energy: Zone 1, Time by Man; or Zone 2, Time by God. Time by Man includes what is important down *here*. Time by God includes only what is important to God, up *there*.

Taxes, money, cars, houses, interest rates, stocks, politics, clothes, lawsuits, position, scores, place, popularity, appearance, and fear are all part of Time by Man.

Charity, love, hope, fairness, honesty, joy, and faith are all characteristics of Time by God.

Wherever your heart and your focus are, your treasure is there also. I want the things of God to be my treasure, not the things of man. When my focus is up and not down, that is when my time and my life are happiest and most abundant.

Spending too much time in Zone 1 being concerned with the needs of the world may sometimes bring you success in the short run, but will only bring you frustration in the long run.

Spending time in Zone 2 being concerned with the needs of God may or may not work out in the short run, but *always* brings success and peace in the long run.

When you begin to live *in the world* but choose not to be part *of the world's* concerns, you no longer absorb trouble in the same way. You will change your point of view and look at the "wants" of God and not the "wants" of the world. You will learn to handle Time by Man with the Time by *God*.

> Do not store up for yourselves treasures on earth, where moth and rust destroy, and where thieves break in and steal. But store up for yourselves treasures in heaven, where moth and rust do not destroy, and where thieves do not break in and steal. For where your treasure is, there your heart will be also. (Matt. 6:19–21)

Do what you are supposed to do . . . (Marvin Lerner)

EMERGENCY-CENTERED LIVING MAKES "MISSION IMPOSSIBLE"

Focusing Your Life on Zone 2 Mission Work

At first glance, most people would look at the two BBG Time Zones and assume they were doing things correctly. After all, this is how they've *always* lived: They are in Zone 1 where they belong and handling emergencies first. Regrettably, *this is not what you are supposed to do.*

When I was a child, I always had a variety of things my parents, teachers, or coaches said I needed to do. Homework, room cleaning, grass mowing, running, or showing up on time were among many of my childhood "assignments." Unhappily, they were also among the many things I never got done. I was always so busy on the phone, playing with my friends, watching TV, going to parties, combing my hair, and trying to get a date that I rarely had time to get anything done.

BBG Owner's Scriptural Guide on Building Strength with Time by God

The rain came down, the streams rose, and the winds blew and beat against that house; yet it did not fall, because it had its foundation on the rock. (Matt. 7:25)

As a result, my grades would be average, weeds would take over the lawn, and my team would lose. Then I would get in trouble, and my father would say, "Do what you're supposed to do!" (Pretty deep if you think about it.)

When you are constantly handling some crisis or tending to another emergency and allowing distractions to rule your life, you have no time left over for what is *really* important. There is always some reason you cannot do what you are "supposed to do."

If you merely spent more time doing what *is* important, you would not have many of these emergencies in the first place, and you most likely wouldn't be getting in trouble for things like failing grades, overgrown lawns, and a losing record.

What is important, what you are supposed to do, is your mission in life. By beginning to focus your life on Time by God Mission Work, many of the emergencies and distractions of Time by Man will begin to disappear, *along with many of your excuses for not doing what you are supposed to do.*

TIME BY GOD IS SPENDING TIME ON MISSION WORK

Time by God in Zone 2 is work you do to advance your mission on earth. It is called "Mission Work." Mission Work encompasses everything it takes to move you and the world forward. This includes the things of God which are uplifting, inspirational, constructive, and empowering.

Time by God Mission Work includes: Healthy Lifestyle, Spiritual Growth, Relationship Building, Skill Sharpening and New Skill Development, Opportunities, Planning and Organization, Social and Community Involvement, Coaching, Maintenance, Perception Reprogramming, and any time spent on these categories Working in Mission.

Mission Work is working *on* your life rather than just reacting to the stress, trouble, and emergencies that are *in* your life.

Healthy Lifestyle

A healthy lifestyle includes any information or activity designed to move you toward your ultimate health potential by maximizing the natural strengths, fitness level, and appearance of your body and its God-given ability to heal. This includes all the *Owner's Manual* plans for better fueling, movement, and stress management.

Spiritual Growth

Spiritual Growth involves time with God. This is time spent praying, listening, and reading in order to move closer to God and cause greater spiritual understanding and growth.

Relationship Building

Prioritize time for family, friends, business associates, and cultural groups on a regular basis in order to create communication, trust, better ideas, teamwork, unity, conflict resolution, and lasting relationships.

Skill Sharpening and New Skill Development

Spend time learning and developing new skills to enhance your value in the areas you are already involved in or becoming effective in new areas. In this type of work, you are enhancing and mastering your skills and abilities so you are always moving toward your God-given potential in all areas of your life.

Opportunities

Seek out and/or *create* personal and business opportunities.

Zone 2 Is the "Peace Management Zone"

Perception Reprogramming is accomplished when you start spending time in self-examination so you can be aware of certain attitudes and behaviors you have that are producing painful outcomes. The goal of perception reprogramming is to change your point of view by evaluating where certain negative thoughts and emotions come from so you can eliminate them at their source and see the world as a more peaceful place.

All activities designed for improved awareness, increased skills, change, and personal growth will work to better your view of the world and the people in it.

Review "Reprogramming Your Perception Software" in the Stress Management section to find out how God can "download" a more heavenly outlook on life.

Planning and Organization

Plan your day, week, month, year, or years in the activities of Zone 2 and organize your life in a schedule to accomplish them.

Social and Community Involvement

Spend time meeting your moral obligations to enhance the community and lighten the burden of others. This is accomplished by working with religious, charitable, fraternal, and other community organizations.

Coaching

Learn and be coached by others who have achieved a higher level of success than you have achieved, particularly in areas you participate in or would like to participate in. You can be coached in sports, business, and relationships with your spouse, with your children, and with God.

Maintenance

Regularly care for your body, your possessions, and your relationships so they continue to function at their optimum level and not break down or need replacing.

20 | MISSION-CENTERED LIVING

Your Mission Is to Be Whatever God Wants You to Be

Growing up, I was always told, "You can be whatever you want to be." At the age of seven, I firmly decided I wanted to be a football player. All through elementary school and on into junior high, if you asked me what I was going to be when I grew up, I would tell you with fervent conviction that I was going to be a football player.

When I reached high school, I was confronted with a glitch in the "you can be whatever you want to be" theory. I was the smallest guy on the high-school football team—by a lot. Although I worked hard and believed enough in myself to manage to make the starting team, it occurred to me that at five-foot-nothing, a hundred and nothing, perhaps I was not created to be a football player.

The alternative was wrestling. God must have specifically created me for that sport because in wrestling, five-foot-nothing-a-hundred-and-nothing people wrestle other five-foot-nothing-a-hundred-and-nothing people. Soon I decided I wanted to make the Olympic Wrestling Team. However, once more I was confronted with physical limitations. I spent more time in doctors' offices getting treated for injuries than I spent practicing or competing. As a result, I had to change directions again.

Eventually I did end up making the Olympic Wrestling Team—as one of their doctors.

Looking back on my life, I have come to realize that as a doctor, a writer, a counselor, and a lecturer, I am able to do far greater things than I ever could have done as an athlete.

God gave me nothing I ever wanted.

Instead, He gave me what the world and I really needed.

The reality is that while you can be whatever you want to be, it also has to be what God created you to be. I wanted to be a famous athlete. Instead, God gave me physical limitations so I could help other people with physical limitations.

That became *my* mission in life . . .

BE YOURSELF, ONLY BETTER

A mission is greater than you are. Rather than being focused on personal wealth, fame, or achievement, a mission is focused around serving God through helping people and the condition of His world.

When you have discovered the mission God has called you to, you find that you have been blessed with strengths and abilities that help you to get the work done. When you are on a mission from God, God aligns all the forces in His universe to work in your favor.

When on your mission, you become yourself, only better.

You have been given a body, a set of skills, specific abilities, and certain passions and desires, all designed to perform your mission. Your mission starts in Zone 2 by building your spirit, strengthening your body, developing your abilities, and mastering your skills. It is only when you do all you can to reach your God-given potential that you can truly serve at the level God has called you to serve. You do not have to reach your potential to serve, but you must reach your potential to serve *your best*. The better you become, the better God can use you.

Being on the right mission may not necessarily mean instant success. If you look at Joseph, Daniel, Moses, John, Jesus, Lincoln, Gandhi, or Martin Luther King, their missions were accompanied by setbacks and tragedies. Nevertheless, God ultimately triumphed and their mission-centered living has gone on to bring hope to millions, glorify God, and affect the way we live and treat each other for all eternity.

No matter what your results appear to be, if your mission is to try to produce the same results as theirs, you, too, are on a "mission from God." When you are on a mission from God, God is with you.

This makes you not only the very best you can be, it makes you even better . . .

MAKING MISSION WORK POSSIBLE

In mission-centered living, you are spending most of your time on Time by God. This entails making mission work the focus of your day. These activities will improve every area of your life and help prevent or eliminate the various troubles, distractions, and emergencies that pull you out of mission-centered living and into emergency-centered living.

BBG Owner's Mission Work List

Healthy Lifestyle, Relationship Building, Spiritual Growth, Social and Community Development, Skill Sharpening and New Skill Development, Opportunities, Planning and Organization, Coaching, Maintenance, Perception Reprogramming, and any time spent on these categories working in mission.

PREVENTING OR ELIMINATING ZONE 1 EMERGENCIES WITH ZONE 2 MISSION-ARY WORK

Time Emergencies	Preventing/Eliminating Emergencies
Zone 1 Emergencies	*Zone 2 Mission-ary Work*
Being late, rushing, missing a plane	Planning and Organization
Doctor visits, pharmacy visits	Healthy Lifestyle, Spiritual Growth, Relationship Building
Counseling, attorney appointments	Relationship Building to prevent family and business crisis, Perception reprogramming
Auto mechanic, repairs	Maintenance of cars and equipment

Relationship Emergencies	Preventing/Eliminating Emergencies
Zone 1 Emergencies	**Zone 2 Mission-ary Work**
Marital counseling, divorce, fights	Relationship Building, Spiritual Growth, Healthy Lifestyle
Child's failing school, conflicts	Healthy Lifestyle, Coaching with other families, parents, and successful parents
Family on drugs	Relationship Building

Personal Emergencies	Preventing/Eliminating Emergencies
Zone 1 Emergencies	**Zone 2 Mission-ary Work**
Overweight, pain and illness, fatigue	Healthy Lifestyle, Spiritual Growth, Coaching
Employment dissatisfaction	Opportunity, Planning and Organization, Skill Sharpening and New Skill Development, Coaching, Spiritual Growth, Healthy Lifestyle
Personality or moral dysfunction	Spiritual Growth, Social and Community Involvement, Coaching
Drinking problem, financial insecurity, lack of or poor relationships, losing things, poor sports performance	Healthy Lifestyle, Spiritual Growth, Skill Sharpening and New Skill Development
Low self-esteem, irritable, depressed	Perception Reprogramming, Coaching

> By feeding your solutions in Zone 2,
> you starve your problems in Zone 1.

PRINCIPLE-DRIVEN BEHAVIOR

All tyrants fall. Therefore, it stands to reason that if you are the opposite of tyrannical, you will rise.

For better or for worse, God holds me to high standards of principled behavior. Not that there have not been an abundant amount of times in the past and still many in the present where my principles didn't stumble; it is just that when they did, I took it on the chin . . . hard! If I play one hand of poker, roll any pair of dice, or do anything else solely for the benefit of making money, I *always* lose! Anytime I do anything of questionable morality, I am caught. Even in elementary school, if ten of us were passing notes in the back of the room, chewing gum in class, or running with scissors, I was the one who always got nailed. I had to write sentences for punishment so many times that even when I wasn't in trouble I would write out, "I will be good to my teacher," or "I will not act up in class" in my spare time so I could keep some on file for when I did have to write them again. Even with my health I have been held to very high standards. In my family, if you don't take care of yourself you die at age fifty. That does not leave much room for error. I learned early on and continue to learn the importance of principled behavior on my prosperity and my future.

While it should seem clear that only good pays off, many people have taken shortcuts, thinking they are getting somewhere quicker, easier, or better. I suppose some people pull that off for a while, but sooner or later catastrophe strikes.

What the world needs now and has always needed is good. Good never goes to waste, and while it may appear to go unnoticed at first, it always pays dividends in the long run. God has always been on the side of and, more important, stays on the side of, men and women with principle.

Principled men and women are those who:

- Do not have a price at which they can be bought.
- Do what is right, not expedient.

- Have a word that is a binding contract.
- Are honest in every transaction, no matter how big or small.
- Make decisions that always take into account the well-being of others.
- Look for a way for everyone to win.
- Believe God is always watching their steps.
- See past what is important in this world and into what is important in God's world.
- Never pay their expenses at the expense of others.
- Passionately desire to be successful in their mission, but will not use deception, cunning, or other people to get there.
- Do not fear rejection, failure, or swimming upstream against popular opinion.
- Are willing to do what has never been done.
- Are inspired to be obedient to doing God's work.
- Are faithful and hopeful.
- Are uncompromising in their leadership.
- Are willing to endure hardships, the tests of time, and do whatever it takes for as long as it takes to see their mission accomplished.

THE LAW OF THE JUNGLE

In the jungle, survival is the law. If you or your family is hungry, threatened, or in need of shelter, you do *whatever it takes* to survive.

Everyone has an innate, Zone 1, desire to survive in the simplest, most readily available way they can. Inborn within us is the instinct to follow the law of the jungle. However, survival is *not* law in a principled life. The law of the principled life is God's Law.

Surviving with "jungle law" is Time by Man zone living. To live in the Time by God zone, you must attempt to handle all life's matters with principle.

We all have the need, and the right, to survive—and more. Total prosperity, including comfortable shelter, good health, pleasurable travel, time with our family, and prosperous financial situations, is the right of all human beings and a gift worthy of achieving. However, none of those things should be achieved at the expense of principle.

Never think that breaking God's law is necessary in order to survive. We can survive in the jungle without becoming animals.

Principle is always your best investment . . .

Survival-Driven Behavior (Jungle Law—Time by Man Zone)	Principle-Driven Behavior (God's Law—Time by God Zone)
Hungry	
Eat (Easiest, tastiest, quickest)	Feed nutritiously (Creates the most: health, energy, healing, leanness)
Money	
My money (Pay bills, get rich)	God's money (Serve a mission)
Decisions	
No one's watching (I must win)	God is always watching (Everyone must win)
Completion	
Now	God's timing—in season, when it's correct
Financial Gain	
To make money—no matter what	Helps others to make money—everything matters
Financial gain (which is an illusion)	With God and fulfilling my mission, I will always be secure (which is a reality)
Effort	
The least resistance possible	Whatever it takes
Time	
Immediate gratification	In God's time—however long it takes

TO ACT (ZONE 2) OR REACT (ZONE 1)? THAT IS THE QUESTION

Day 1: Drove down a street and crashed into a tree.

Day 2: Drove down the same street and crashed into the same tree.

Day 3: Drove down the same street and crashed into the same tree.

Day 4: Drove down the same street and crashed into the same tree.

Day 5: Drove down a different street.

I counseled a very nice but sad woman who told me she had three children who turned out the way every parent fears. All three of her children had problems with using illegal drugs, had dropped out of school, had multiple divorces, and were always out of work. She wanted some advice from me because she had become responsible for taking care of some of her grandchildren and they were heading in the same direction.

I immediately began to think cause-actively (Zone 2). I came to the conclusion that since every child this poor lady took care of turned out wrong, then there must be something she was doing to cause it.

Sadly, she was thinking reactively (Zone 1). When I asked her why she thought that her children and grandchildren had so much trouble in life, she blamed circumstance. She felt she had good kids and had done a great job raising them, but that the school, the neighborhood, the guidance counselors, and others had all failed them in some way.

As it turns out, I discovered what was most likely the real problem: When her children got in trouble, she did what she thought every loving mother would do—she got them out of trouble. Never once did one of her children have to deal with the consequences of their own bad behavior. In fact, when I asked her what punishment they received at home for what must have been countless serious offenses, she said that she believed in showing love and understanding and not punishing.

She was now doing exactly the same thing with her grandchildren and expecting a different result. She was going to drive down the same street and expect not to crash into the same tree.

I told her that waiting until problems develop and then trying to figure out the best way to solve them or blaming the environment and those around her for her problems is being reactive and living in Zone 1. I told her it was time to start living in Zone 2 and become cause-active. It was time to start acting in a way to cause her grandchildren not to take drugs, to develop good learning skills, and to understand godly ways.

This would cause them to turn out well.

I further explained to her that her grandchildren had to face the repercussions of immorality, lack of education, and unemployment. I wanted her grandchildren to see what happens when you place the wrong "causes" in motion in your life before it is too late.

If a parent wants a child to grow up well, but waits until things go wrong, then gets upset and starts blaming bad luck and everyone around them, then that parent is being reactive.

That is a Zone 1 focus.

If a parent wants a child to grow up the right way, he or she must set all the right *causes* in motion throughout the child's life to help *create* those effects. They need to cause-actively create a positive outcome.

That is Zone 2 focus.

**Reactive people ask what is wrong with the world;
cause-active people ask what they can do to change the world.**

Zone 2 focus allows you to be more at *cause* in your life. The world is filled with challenges and bumpy roads that you and those you love may end up driving down, no matter what you do. Still, Zone 2 cause-action rather than Zone 1 reaction will give you your best chance at a smoother ride.

BBG Owner's Power Tip: The Law of Cause and Effect

Results are an effect, you are the cause. If you choose to cause-actively create positive results, then you are the cause of the victory. If you do nothing and you lose, you are the cause of defeat.

Either way, *you* are the cause.

You are a cause in your life, not an effect. Don't wait for the world to change around you and cause life to get better. Change yourself in the world around you to cause life to get better.

Change yourself, and you change the world.

PERFECT PRAYER

In essence, prayer is being cause-active at creating better results in your life. Prayer works. Even scientific research has proved it. And because God can do *anything,* sometimes prayer is all it takes.

However, do not ask God for financial security and keep spending twice what you make. Do not pray for good health but continue to eat Food by Man, exercise annually, be stressed out, and take a lot of medication. Do not pray for a better relationship and not become a better person *in* a relationship.

Perfect prayer is praying to God with total faith that He is able and willing to create the outcome you desire and then doing everything you are supposed to be cause-actively doing in your Time by God to help *create* the outcome you desire.

If you do not get the things you work and pray for, you can still be cause-active in your attitude and your perceptions. If you are alone, in pain, in financial trouble, or dealing with a difficult child, you can still choose whether to be hopeful and have faith that your situation will improve or be reactive and choose to be lonely, afraid, and frustrated.

Pray as if everything depends on God, but work (Mission Work) as though everything depends on you.

CAUSE-ACTIVELY TAKING CHARGE OF MY PROBLEMS LED TO TOTAL OFFICE SOLUTIONS

When I first opened my practice, I had trouble keeping employees. I blamed my location for producing people that lacked work ethic, responsibility, and commitment. As a result of my employee situation, my office was always in an administrative crisis.

Finally, as I was once again blaming other people and my environment for my circumstances, it occurred to me that maybe my business skills were lacking. I began to realize that I was most likely the root cause of my problems.

With my new realization I went out and received some coaching, did some skill sharpening and new skill development, learned how to properly plan and organize my office, and prayed—a lot. Soon things came under control. By cause-actively taking charge of my situation and focusing my time on Zone 2: Mission Work, instead of reacting to Zone 1: Emergencies, my troubles shrank and my solutions began to grow.

To prove the power of Zone 2 living, I eventually started a seminar and consulting company that teaches others about hiring, staff training, organization, and practice management. Whatever your problem is, Time by God will almost always be the solution.

TIME THIEVES WILL BE PROSECUTED!

Like Robin Hood robbing from the rich and giving to the poor, Zone 1 distractions rob *time* from Time by God and give it to Time by Man. World events, news, other people's behaviors, problems, and opinions, personal challenges, mail, e-mail, cell phones, pagers, beepers, TV, fringe businesses, amusing hobbies, regrets, worries, concerns, and allowing yourself to get sick and needing visits to the medical doctor are all voracious time thieves. You cannot afford to be robbed by these "thieves of time" on a regular basis.

While certain distractions can be entertaining and some distractions and "downtimes" are necessary to give your brain a break, these time thieves can steal countless important hours out of your week and severely stunt your emotional and personal growth and prosperity.

For your protection and for the good of humankind, time thieves *must* be treated with extreme prejudice and, if necessary, put away for life!

OBEDIENCE IS FREEDOM?

The obedience to perform work that serves your mission sounds tough. Many people look at the guidelines in this *Owner's Manual* as a lawful, dry, and boring existence. But it is not.

Far from it . . .

The life that is inspired and obedient to God is the blessed life. It is a life that goes beyond simple happiness into an inner sense of peace and fulfillment that can be given to you only by God. It is true, permanent joy and absolute, total freedom.

Schedule your time—and become free!

21 | SCHEDULING A BETTER LIFE

Painting Solid Yellow Lines Around Time by God

There is always enough time to get the important things done. The problem is never truly that there is not enough time; the problem is that there is not enough time *management*.

I have multiple areas of my life that I consider to be firmly planted in Time by God. It is critical to me that each of these areas be done well. In order to do this, I have to look at myself as almost having split personalities. I literally have seven lives:

1. Spiritual Life
2. Family Life
3. Personal Health-and-Fitness Life
4. Patient-Care Life
5. Author Life
6. Lecturer Life
7. Consultant Life

All these lives help others and serve God, so each is worthy of being done with excellence. All my lives together make up my mission. I am passionate about each area and do not look at any area as work, but as loving, joyful, blessed service.

> ### Time is abundant, and when you take from abundance, you still have abundance.

There is a saying: "If you want something done, give it to a busy person." I have changed that to "If you want something done well, give it to a busy, successful person." Busy, successful people have learned how to compartmentalize their time so they can get *multiple* things done better than many people can get *one* thing done.

It would be easy to look at my many lives and say I must be overworked and miserable. Not that I never am. Who isn't overworked and miserable at some point in their lives? But it is not very often. Through proper compartmentalization and delegation, my life is actually fun and fairly easy to manage.

Paint Lines

The important thing is to draw lines around each life. When you are driving, if there is a dotted yellow line, you can pass or cross over into the other lane. However, if there is a solid yellow line, you cannot pass and you cannot cross over. Others cannot pass or cross over either. I paint solid yellow lines around each of my lives and the Mission Work they contain. That way, other lives cannot pass or cross over, and I cannot pass or cross over into them.

For example, on Monday morning I have my Spiritual Life, my Author Life, and my Patient Care Life. In order for me to accomplish all three of these important lives successfully, I must create focused time for *each one*.

From 5:00 A.M. to 6:00 A.M. is my Spiritual Life. At that time I am nothing else. I draw a solid yellow line next to that life so I am not a doctor, author, or speaker. During this period of time, I am a student of the Bible and a prayer warrior and nothing else. No other life is allowed in at that time. I do not take calls, the kids aren't up yet (hopefully), and I do not look at any e-mail.

At 6:00 A.M., my Author Life starts. There is a solid yellow line between Spiritual Life and Author Life. Once it hits 6:00 A.M., Spiritual Life time cannot cross over, and Author Life time cannot cross back. (Although the time you spend on your spiritual life goes with you everywhere.) Author Life goes from 6:00 A.M. to 6:45 A.M. with total concentration on writing.

At 6:45 A.M. I become a doctor. There is another solid yellow line drawn between Author Life and Doctor Life. I drive to my office and see patients from 7:30 A.M. to 11:00 A.M. At 11:00 A.M., you guessed it, another solid yellow line is drawn and I begin another life. Sometimes it's nap life—but it's still scheduled. I learned that one in kindergarten.

Each day has Spiritual Life, Family Life, and Health Life. All my other lives are strategically placed throughout the week so all that needs to be accomplished is done *well*.

Obviously, it doesn't always work out so perfectly. Sometimes a child wakes up during times designated for reading or an extremely urgent issue pops up that cannot be handled by the people to whom I have delegated authority. At those times, I have to practice flexibility. I do not want to become massively stressed when something or someone tries to get by me in the "no passing lane."

If lives "cross over" into other lives, as they occasionally will, I try to remember the admonition "That's life." I work to get past the issues and try to get everyone and everything back in their lanes as quickly as possible before there is an accident!

Unfortunately, a few times a year there are some traumatic, stressful five-life pileups. But by getting back to proper compartmentalization through the painting of solid yellow lines and proper delegation, I usually manage to escape with only some minor damage.

BBG Owner's Time Management Tip: Moment Management

At the age of fifty-two, my father died suddenly and without warning. The unexpected shock of his death and his early departure from the planet left me feeling bitter for a couple of years. What finally got me past the feeling that I had been shortchanged or somehow ripped off was looking back on my life and realizing that I'd had a lot of good "moments" with my dad over the time of his short life.

My father was your classic late-twentieth-century working dad. Even though he was gone before I got up for school and came home late for dinner every night, I always had tremendous respect and appreciation for him.

I respected how hard he worked, that he was great at his job, and that he had reached several positions of authority. I appreciated the fact that, although we were not rich, we never wanted for anything. When he walked in the door at the end of the day, my little brothers and I were not just happy to see him, we were jumping out of our skin, bouncing off of the walls.

As hard as my father worked, and as focused as he was, never for a second did I feel neglected. The reason I always felt loved and appreciated was that while most of his week was consumed by work, when we were together we had endless good "moments."

I truly do not remember being without my dad, but I totally remember everything about being with my dad. The games, the catches, the wrestling matches, the car rides, vacations, movies, meals, lectures about life, and the time when I was in college and he drove four hours to surprise me at a bus station so I wouldn't have to take the bus home, are all "moments" that are indelibly carved into my brain and my spirit forever.

The quality of your life is not measured by the amount of time you spend, it is measured by the amount of "moments" you have in it. You should have many "lives," Business Life, Purpose Life, Spiritual Life, Student Life, Husband/Wife/Boy or Girlfriend Life, and Dad or Mom Life. The quality and effectiveness of these "lives" will be determined by the focus and energy you put into the "moments" within these "lives" rather than just the time you spend on them.

I don't feel cheated out of time with my dad. The fact that he worked a lot or died too soon does not bother me. When I reflect back on my childhood and early adulthood, I thank God for the many incredible "moments" He allowed my dad and me to share before He took my dad home. I don't blame Him; I'd want my dad home too!

DELEGATION ADDS EVEN MORE TIME

Many of my lives have details I delegate to someone else. I don't cut my grass, build my own deck, fix anything that breaks, order supplies at my office, do my own taxes, or change my own oil. The more world-zone activities and God-zone details I can pass on to someone else, the more time I have for my Mission Work.

Delegation also dramatically speeds up results. Not only am I more effective at the life I am living, but there are several other people helping me to move the other lives I have *forward*. So while I am being an author, a team of people are helping my lecture series grow and my clinic run smoothly.

All the people I delegate to have my schedule so they know when they can call me. People helping me with the details of my Author Life know to leave a message or e-mail me when I am in my Doctor Life. We speak or meet at set times throughout the week that are designated Author Life times. The accountants and managers in charge of business issues send me daily and weekly reports and updates to keep me abreast of what is happening. I then read these items and/or meet with these people only during designated Business Life times weekly or monthly.

If someone helping me with my Lecturer Life tries to contact me when I am in my Family Life or someone from my Business Life tries to call me when I am in my Author Life, I let the voice mail get it or have someone take a message. I wait until I am back in my Lecturer Life or Business Life to return those calls or handle those issues.

When I first try to get people to start delegating, I usually run into two problems:

Problem #1: The Control Freak

Many people have some control issues, but most people have *huge* control issues. At some point in your life, you are going to have to trust somebody if you are ever going to take some weight off your back, reduce your stress, and move forward. Issues dealing with money, family, and important areas of your home or business may be hard for you to "let go" of, but you must learn to delegate even the vital things. It may take considerable time and prayer to find the right type of person, but there are a lot of high-quality, trustworthy people who need good jobs and would love to help you achieve your mission.

Problem #2: Penny-Smart and Dollar-Dumb

Understanding cost versus investment is another major reason people refuse to delegate. I hear things like: "Why should I pay someone to mow my lawn (clean my house, paint my fence, do my taxes) when I can just do it myself?" This is called being "penny-wise and dollar-dumb." You save pennies and cost yourself thousands. While you are busy picking up socks, trimming hedges, and putting Armor-All on your tires, you could be advancing your skills, growing your business, playing with your kids, or supporting your religious organization. You can easily spend several hundred hours a year working on "stuff" and "details" that you could have paid only pennies to someone else to accomplish for you. You could have used all that time to exponentially explode your life and construct a future to be proud of.

There are plenty of neighbors' kids who will cut your lawn for twenty dollars. If you cut your own lawn, you steal that kid's twenty dollars. You also steal time away from God, your family, and yourself.

> Two are better than one, because they have a good return for their work: If one falls down, his friend can help him up. But pity the man who falls and has no one to help him up! (Eccl. 4:9–10)

YOUR SOLID YELLOW LINES HELP YOU LIVE A LIFE OF EXCELLENCE

When departmentalizing your life, you must create maximum-security, impenetrable barriers between lives.

When I am an author, I am focused on being an author and not a doctor. When I am a doctor, I am focused on being a doctor and not an author *or* a lecturer. When I am a family man, I am focused on being a family man and not an author, a doctor, *or* a lecturer. This guarantees not only living these lives, but living them with excellence.

The scheduling forms at the end of the chapter are a very generalized view of a typical day during the week doing what it takes to lead many lives with focus and excellence. In between some of these times are things like food, some enjoyable reading, movies, and some phone calls with close friends. While life should run by the hour, it would be tough and somewhat restrictive to have it run by the minute or the second.

The people I delegate to carry out many of the details, production, and promotion of my lives also have compartmentalized times for their work throughout the week that are blocked out with solid yellow lines.

At designated times throughout the day, week, or month, I meet or speak with the people I have delegated items to or read and answer their e-mails to me. These activities have solid yellow lines around them as well.

When planning your time, God is first, your family is second, and your mission is third.

Through compartmentalizing my life by painting solid yellow lines and delegating a tremendous amount of work, I have become very time efficient. I can live out my multiple lives with passion, excellence, and considerable productivity.

On the other hand, while I am very efficient with *time,* I am careful not to be efficient with *God or people.* As a husband, dad, doctor, and someone who is always seeking God, I have to constantly remind myself that God and other people come first. Particularly the people closest to me whom I have the opportunity and responsibility to help. Therefore, I can never become subdued into thinking I am too busy achieving to stop and show my love and appreciation to God and the people who need *me.*

God must be your *first* love. To show love for God, it is important to consider what He wants. I imagine God wants what most fathers would want. (Remember, this is your heavenly Father, so what He wants does not include more time fishing or lying on the couch watching football.) A father wants you to love Him, spend time with Him, and not get caught up in the bad things and useless distractions of the world. The Bible's word on this topic states, "Do not love the world or anything in the world. If anyone loves the world, the love of the Father is not in him" (1 John 2:15).

Home Delegation

My wife, Dr. Sheri, runs a large chiropractic clinic, is a mom, and has a very active fitness and spiritual life. We delegate parenting and other family responsibilities to each other whenever possible so we can both get our "lives" accomplished.

When our schedules clash at times, we delegate and get a baby-sitter or a grandma to help. We do this even if it is just a half hour to let her get a workout in or to be there if my wife and I want to pray or go for a run together.

For the success of your family and to help find prosperity in all areas, be sure to delegate at home.

The Only Life I Always Lead (I Am Third)

1. God

2. Family

3. Me

That is why my Spiritual Life is always the first life I lead in the morning and Family Life is a daily priority.

The people I work with or deal with every day are not a means to an end. I do all that I can to lead and encourage them and not just get something from them.

You can be efficient and economical with time, but you must be helpful and effective with people. *In every life you lead, God comes first, your family comes second, and you are third.*

BBG Owner's Emergency Protection Plan

By blocking out days and daily times for God and family life, you help to prevent many of the emergencies that would cross over the yellow lines into your other lives.

GENERALIZED TIME CHART—DR. BEN LERNER

MORNING/AFTERNOON

Time: 5–6 A.M.	Time: 6–6:45 A.M.	Time: 6:45–11 A.M.	Time: 11 A.M.–1 P.M.	Time: 1–1:45 P.M.
Life: Spiritual	Life: Author	Life: Doctor	Life: Consultant	Life: Health

AFTERNOON/EVENING

Time: 2–6 P.M.	Time: 6–9 P.M.	Time: 9–10 P.M.	Time: 10 P.M.	Time:
Life: Doctor	Life: Family	Life: Lecturer	Life: Sleep	Life:

(SYL)   (SYL)   (SYL)   (SYL)   (SYL)

SOLID YELLOW LINE (SYL)

GENERALIZED PERSONAL TIME CHART

MORNING/AFTERNOON

Time:	Time:	Time:	Time:	Time:
Life:	Life:	Life:	Life:	Life:

AFTERNOON/EVENING

Time:	Time:	Time:	Time:	Time:
Life:	Life:	Life:	Life:	Life:

(SYL) (SYL) (SYL) (SYL)

SOLID YELLOW LINE (SYL)

PART SIX | LIFE BY GOD

22 | APPLYING YOUR MISSION WORK

Time by God Is Life by God

Remember, your body is by God, for God, and is God's. A true Life by God is a life in which you have discovered your gifts, are satisfied in your work, take care of your Body by God, enjoy loving relationships, and experience peace—whatever your circumstance. Life by God is total prosperity; success in not just one, but in all of the important areas of your life.

This elusive, mystical, and prosperous Life by God I speak of is possible through loving God so much that you are inspired (See Rule #4 of the Four Rules of Olympic Success) to the point of obedience to Time by God Mission Work.

However difficult or challenging Mission Work appears to be at first, over time, you will reap such unbelievable benefits from living a Life by God that you will not be able to imagine living life any other way. Remember, Mission Work fits within your passion and your calling and supports the things you do that serve God, your family, and the world. Eventually, on the days you do nothing to support your "mission from God," you will miss it badly.

> *For we are God's fellow workers; you are God's field, God's building. (1 Cor. 3:9)*

BBG Owner's Power Tip

Focusing your life on Time by God is making your life God's life. This is a very powerful, low-stress way to live.

See "The 10 Instructions for Peace by God" and look under Instruction #8: Thou Shalt Be Fearless (page 272)—"It's God's Life, Not Yours" for more on what making your life God's life can do for you.

BBG OWNER'S PROSPERITY TIMES GUIDE

Time by God Mission Work contains "Prosperity Times" that support it. These Prosperity Times work to help you discover, develop, and express your gifts so you may better carry out your mission and live a Life by God.

Healthy Lifestyle and Spiritual Growth have more "Special Times" than any other form of Mission Work. These "Special Times" are the most important part of a Life by God because they allow for better performance and results in all areas of life and in the other forms of Mission Work. You take them with you wherever you go.

Many people know *of* God, but few people actually *know* God. Spiritual Growth times are times with God. The more time you spend with Him, the more you get to know Him and love Him. Sooner or later, you will find that time with God is not only your most productive time of day, it is your favorite time of day.

While some of the Special Times you spend during Healthy Lifestyle or Spiritual Growth Mission Work may seem as though you are doing nothing, the impact they have in every part of your life actually ends up making them the most fruitful part of your day.

Healthy Lifestyle

Aerobic Time. For optimum cardiovascular and physiological health and function, it is vital that you set up a minimum of two to three aerobic-movement activities a week for a minimum of fifteen to twenty minutes each. These can be set up as simply FUR movements only or a combination of FUR/PER/SUR, if you wish to become more athletic or competitive.

See the Exercise by God section of your Owner's Manual for directions for setting up and performing aerobic-movement routines.

Resistance Time. A minimum of two Exercise by God resistance movement programs are necessary for maintaining healthy muscle-to-body-fat ratios in order to prevent disease.

See the Exercise by God section of your Owner's Manual for directions for setting up and performing resistance-movement routines.

Nutrition Time. Following through on a solid Food by God nutrition program takes planning, shopping time, and food-preparation time. Special nutrition time must be set aside and protected each week, or even each day, if you are going to stop eating what's easiest and start eating what God intended you to eat.

See the Food by God section of your *Owner's Manual* to review the Un-Diet—eating Food by God according to the Un-Diet Food Guide.

Spiritual Growth

Quiet Time. Western society often looks at other cultures that live in poverty or who exist without videos, cell phones, Internet, movie theaters, nice houses, cars, restaurants, and all the other "modern" essentials of an "advanced" civilization and wonders how they do it.

On the contrary, people in many less "advanced" cultures look at our "modern" society and wonder how we do it. They wonder how people could live in cities with all the noise, distractions, and without as much real evidence of the presence of God.

Modern society is a loud concrete jungle. Most worlds are now filled with TV, radios, and masses of people driving and walking down paved roads and sidewalks in commercial and housing developments that used to be fields and forests. This "modern" and "advanced" living allows for no quiet, peaceful time in nature. This makes it very difficult to really hear, see, and, especially, *feel* the presence of God.

God is always with you. When you are in the silence, you are more likely to also be with Him. At least one time per day, usually early in the morning, it is important to find a quiet place in nature or at least designate a special, relaxing place in your home for Quiet Time. Stay in the silence for as long as possible. Even though you are in a quiet place, it may be difficult at first for you to relax and shut off your "brain noise."

In order to reach a silent, meditative state, focus on deep, slow breaths. Breathe in and fill your stomach, and breathe out through your chest. When you breathe in, your stomach goes out. When you breathe out, your chest goes out. After you breathe in, hold for two to four times longer than it took you to breathe in. Then breathe out for two times longer than it took you to breathe in.

This focus on your breathing will not only super-oxygenate your BBG, it will also distract your mind and slow down or even stop the internal dialogue that can be so distracting to your time with God. Eventually, you will begin to enjoy the silence more and more and stay there longer with better effects. Soon, you will not know how you ever lived without it.

Bible Time. Quiet Time is for hearing what God says. Bible Time is for reading what God says. All the best ways of attaining peace, building solid relationships, and handling life's challenges are written in the Bible. When accepted in full faith, the Bible is a source of power for all good, bad, and indifferent times.

Many of the examples, metaphors, and illustrations necessary to a less stressful, more productive life are in the Bible. Do not wait until you encounter difficult times and *then* begin searching out God for answers. Seek Him first by spending time reading the Bible each day.

Choose a time or even several times each day for reading. Like Quiet Time, Bible Time may also be challenging at first. However, soon the Book will be a great source of enjoyment for you, and you will clearly see how it helps you down the road of success.

Prayer Time. Quiet Time was for listening, Bible Time was for reading, and Prayer Time is for talking to God. This is a time to ask Him questions, and to ask that His will be done through you. There is power in the spoken word. Going to your Father and talking to Him, as if He is alive and real, which He is, is a major way of building your faith and getting results in your life.

Pray for your family and friends and *with* your family and friends. Pray for your town, your state, your country, and their leaders. Pray for the poor, the sick, and the needy. Pray for your enemies and those who live without God. Pray that in all things you and others do, God will be there, offer protection, and that His will may be done.

*And pray in the Spirit on **all** occasions with all kinds of prayers and requests.* (Eph. 6:18, emphasis added)

Life by God Booster #1: Go to Bed Early

God is first. He is supposed to get your best fruit. Therefore, God should get the best of your day and not some little part left over before bedtime or at the end of the week. How would your spouse, your girlfriend, or your boyfriend feel if you met with them only on Sundays for a couple of hours and then said, "Great seein' ya again; catch ya next Sunday"?

I have found the only way I can get consistent, good-quality time with God and truly give Him my best is if I do it first thing in the morning. That way God gets the time before my day, as well as everyone else's day, starts or takes off.

I get up early enough every morning to accomplish the "Spiritual Triathlon": some quiet (listening) time, Bible (reading) time, and some prayer (speaking) time. The morning time is God's time. If I schedule it for later, it won't have the same intensity, and it may not even happen. God time also puts me in the right state of mind so I write, speak, and work with patients more effectively.

I do not consider myself a morning person. In fact, although my morning time is focused around Spiritual Growth, the first person to speak to me in the morning is not God, it's the devil. The first thing I hear is, "Hit the snooze button" or "Go back to sleep. God knows you could really use another half hour." I do not typically hear, "Wahoo! Five o'clock in the morning, my favorite time of day!"

The first step in managing morning wake-ups is to get to bed in time to get between seven and a half to eight hours of sleep. This is accomplished the same way as everything else in a Life by God. You need to paint solid yellow lines around bedtime. That way, when Satan speaks first in the morning, you can give him the appropriate answer: "Shut up!"

"Be still, and know that I am God" (Ps. 46:10).

Thank Him for everything, good or bad, and make prayer time the best part or the fruit of your day, and not just a piece left over at the end. Pray when you wake up, pray before meals, pray before work, pray before interacting with people, and not just a quickie prayer before you go to bed that you learned to recite in nursery school.

Organized Worship Time. Visiting a place of worship on a consistent basis on a specific day is key to receiving joy and peace from God. Structured worship taught by experienced religious professionals will bring about greater understanding of the Bible and help you to strengthen your relationship with God.

The group dynamic of a religious organization further brings the support and accountability necessary to follow through on your spiritual life.

Inspirational Time. Along with being educational, certain books, audios, videos, and speakers can be inspirational. Exposing yourself and your family to inspirational multimedia versus the many other types of negative materials that are available keeps you and those around you positive and inspired.

Relationship Building

Date Time. To avoid the stress of relationship emergencies, time in the principal's office, and the pain and expense of corporate and divorce attorneys, it is critical to work on building your relationships frequently with your spouse, children, girl-/boyfriend, relatives close friends, and important business associates.

Pick a morning, afternoon, or evening and schedule a special time with the people who are important to you. Each person gets his or her own date and time. People like your spouse and children get a date time at the same or similar time every week with a solid yellow line surrounding—and protecting—it.

Life by God Booster #2: Keep the Fire Burning with Date Time

For a fire to survive, the logs cannot stand alone. Logs burn longer, brighter, and hotter when they are surrounded by other logs. An incredibly important part of your week in which to spend committed, compartmentalized energy is in the building of your relationships. All health and peace will fail if your relationships are falling apart, and no money or success is as important as the people in your world.

Few of us spend near as much time building our basic human relationships as we should. As a result, we lose a lot of time and sleep dealing with *relationship emergencies*. Relationship emergencies can become the most stressful part of our existence and will completely debilitate any chance at having a Life by God.

Relationship emergencies usually come from a lack of communication. For instance: There is a young married couple who have not communicated enough due to the brevity of their relationship and the fact that they are both very busy with work. One night, the young man comes home late, goes to get a drink of water and sees that there is a glass in the sink that his wife left there three days ago. He then thinks to himself that she does that all the time and he really hates that. Tired and in a bad mood, he chooses right then to ask his wife why she does not put glasses in the dishwasher after she uses them.

Realizing she always does that and he must have been unhappy with this for months, she gets very upset and decides to tell him about a thing or two she hates. The end result is a massive relationship emergency due to lack of communication.

Relationship building/communication times with business partners, employees, relatives, friends, spouses, children, etc., are vital parts in your week to paint solid yellow lines around. This will stop marriages and business relationships from going from the honeymoon to the courtroom, keep your kids out of counseling and principals' offices, and help you continue to get invited to your aunt's house for Thanksgiving.

The best way to assure regular interaction with the people in your life who are important to you is to schedule *date times*. Date times are time slots you etch in stone at some point each week, morning, afternoon, or night, when you and someone with whom you wish to build and maintain a solid, committed relationship can enjoy some time together.

Your spouse and individual children get time each week, and your close friends, relatives, and important business associates get time at least monthly.

Each child and adult should get his or her own date time. Do not put them all in a room one day a week and call it "mission accomplished."

Date times are things like breakfast out with your spouse right after the kids are dropped off at school every Tuesday morning, your child's favorite movie or video every Thursday night, dinner with your best friend or important business associate every third Monday at 7:00 P.M., or a call to your aunt in Alaska every Friday at noon!

Though one may be overpowered, two can defend themselves. (Eccl. 4:12)

Social and Community

Charitable Time. Helping your community and contributing to organizations that have the purpose of assisting the needy in your area make you active in improving your environment. While others feel helpless and victimized and fear how terrible the world has gotten, Charitable Time will make you feel powerful as you cause the world to improve.

Skill Sharpening and New Skill Development

Educational Time. Time spent learning the latest technology in your area of expertise, expanding your knowledge base to new areas of proficiency, and exposing yourself to information on how to live a peaceful, successful, and purposeful life make up Educational Time.

This time of personal growth and self-empowerment is critical to your continued spiritual growth and maturity. Time alone does not create growth, Educational Time does. Otherwise, the older people got, the happier they would be, and this is usually not the case.

Committing to finish books, audios, and videos, signing up for classes and seminars, and scheduling coaching and masterminding time should be a consistent part of your schedule.

Continue to get better at what you do, and learn to do new things. The world is ever advancing. The number-one reason for failure in business, health, *and* relationships is simply "staying the same."

Only the mediocre think they are always at their best. You are either growing or dying. Putting time into sharpening your skills and developing new proficiencies will keep you on top of things and better able to adapt to a constantly developing world.

Life by God Booster #3: Getting Undistracted

There is such a thing as spending too much time wasting time. In fact, I know some people who go through their mail and read all the junk mail along with all the vital mail. It's plainly junk, and yet they read it from cover to cover anyway. Same with their e-mails, cell phones, pager messages, and other distractions. They answer every call right away, along with all their crucial business and family calls. I've seen them spend hours doing that—precious, vital hours—and then complain in the same breath about not having enough hours in the day!

Naturally, few people have enough time to waste even a precious second of it. Wasting time causes you to miss out on a tremendous amount of opportunities. So be careful to spend your time wisely, and never, ever waste it. Prioritize what it will take to bring abundance and peace to the important areas of your life and focus your time there. Put off, get rid of, or delegate distracting time wasters that do not help you create prosperity in your life.

Opportunities

Launching Time. Going forth into the personal and business communities and exposing yourself to more of what is out there will give you the potential to find new opportunities and be upwardly mobile in *all* areas of your life.

After all, if you don't get the bat off your shoulder, how will you ever be a hit? Opportunity Time is not waiting for your ship to come in, it is launching your own ship.

Planning and Organization

Playbook Time. Your plan, your playbook, or your "life map" is critical to winning or ending up exactly where you desire to go. Planning the methods and strategies necessary to make changes and achieve necessary outcomes is paramount to your prosperity or success in every part of your life.

Life by God Booster #4: Forget to Plan, Then Plan to Forget

The reason they call it time "management" is because the word *management* implies some direct action that needs to be taken in order for your time to be actively "managed." For instance, to increase the need for repetitive physical movement or activity in your life, you don't just try to "squeeze in a workout" if time permits or you remember.

That is not managing your time; that is time managing you.

That is "managing" to let yourself off the hook when deadlines loom, meetings go late, you get hungry and tired, or forget and zoom past the gym on your way home. That is not cause-acting to make things happen in the Time by God Zone, that is reacting so things almost never happen in the Time by Man zone.

If you want to start exercising regularly, you must cause-actively say, "At six in the morning on Monday, at five in the afternoon on Tuesday, and at six on Saturday night, I am exercising. That's it. Period. End of story." That way, you cause exercise to happen. It gets written in the book, and it's a done deal. Now you won't forget, and you'll stick to that plan.

You are finally managing your time.

Need to start eating better? Then don't start the week without some preparation. If you do, you will end up stuck at lunch and suddenly it's an emergency. You are starving, and the "Law of the Jungle" sets in, and all you are thinking about now is survival. The only place around that you have time for is a fast-food chain or a convenience store, and instead of causing yourself to eat healthy, you end up reacting to your hunger emergency.

If you are going to start eating better, you have to plan it. You have to manage your time in order to find the time to make things work. You go shopping every Sunday, you cook for two or three days at a time instead of one meal at a time, and you put some healthy food in containers that you can take to work with you. Then, when you are hungry, you already have healthy food right there next to you, and you can skip the candy bar or the cheeseburger.

You can't just try to figure out Mission Work when you get to it or try to remember it as you go. No matter what your situation, you need to start planning. Put it in the schedule, and stick to the schedule.

Goal-Setting Time. Without goals, you are traveling without a compass *or* a destination. You have to be consciously focused on a bull's-eye in order to achieve your desired results. Set apart time every week, month, and year for organizing your goals.

Setting and resetting goals is as important to your survival and success as it is to breathe in and out. Writing down goals is also a tremendous act of faith. It shows that you are believing in God to bring the very things He has placed in your heart to write down. Remember, faith is the substance of things hoped for, so write down your goals and have faith that they are as real as the pen you are writing with or the seat you are sitting in.

See "The 10 Instructions for Peace by God" and look under Instruction #9: Thou Shalt Be Faithful—"It's Not What You Know, It's Who You Are."

Life by God Booster #5: Don't Smudge Your Lines

Show me a winner without goals, and I will show you an eventual loser.

Show me a loser with goals, and I will show you an eventual winner.

A great athlete, coach, teacher, carpenter, accountant, painter, doctor, student, landscaper, spouse, parent, or great *anything* has goals. Anyone with a future also has goals. No goals, no greatness, no future.

It is vitally important that you always have multiple, up-to-date goals. Setting specific goals in all the important areas of your life and then setting an even more specific plan for how to achieve each one of them will assure some level of, if not total, *prosperity.*

Start by writing down, in detail, all your dreams and everything you want to accomplish in your time here on this planet. Then be extraspecific in writing down your plan for how you will go about achieving each goal. Leave no detail unwritten on what it would take for your dreams to be fulfilled.

When following your plan, commit to doing each of the things you wrote down exactly as written. *Do not smudge your lines!* If you said you were going to jog a mile, three times per week, then jog a mile, three times per week. If you said you were going to make ten sales calls a day, then make at least ten sales calls per day. Do not skip or shortchange any part of your plan. If you do, you put reaching your goals in jeopardy.

All goals need to be written down and verbalized. There is amazing, supernatural power in the written and spoken word. This will hold you accountable for achieving them. Your coaches, mentors, and people in your mastermind group are great for helping you to choose, formulate, reformulate, and stick to your plans for reaching your goals.

Each time you reach a goal, write "God's Victory" next to the goal. In addition, have a victory party in honor of your achievement and give yourself a special gift. (Writing down goals and plans works, so try to make your gifts CDs and hiking trips in the mountains rather than pizza and cheesecake. This way, you do not end up needing the additional goal of having to drop a hundred pounds by the time you've reached the rest of your goals!)

Coaching

Masterminding Time. Masterminding means meeting with people who have goals and beliefs similar to yours so you may reap the benefits of the wisdom of others as well as the benefits of a team effort toward meeting those goals.

Life by God Booster #6: Sharpen the Ax

There is no great athlete, composer, business leader, or religious leader who did not have a great teacher. The fastest, least painful way to the top is to have someone show you the quickest, easiest way.

I have coaches for everything. I have spiritual coaches, marriage coaches, health coaches, parenting coaches, financial coaches, sports coaches, and business coaches. Rarely do I make important decisions in my life without consulting some of these people.

My coaches are also the people I spend my time with. These are the people with whom I choose to eat dinner and go on vacation. I do this because when I am with them I am made a better person. These people sharpen my ax. They make me more capable of moving through life as a sharpened ax is able to move through wood—cleaner, easier, and more effectively.

I don't even personally know some of my coaches. They are authors, lecturers, and business leaders. I go to their seminars, listen to their tapes, and study their organizations as a way of continuing to motivate myself and get even sharper.

"If the ax is dull and its edge unsharpened, more strength is needed but skill will bring success" (Eccl. 10:10).

Maintenance

Prevention Time. Maintaining mechanical and technical equipment is crucial to avoiding many emergencies. Spending time without transportation due to a broken-down car, waiting in repair shops, or going to the store to replace equipment is incredibly stressful and can be entirely avoided with proper maintenance of your possessions. While taking care of your things may seem hard or time-consuming while you are doing it, it will be easier, less stressful, and timesaving in the long run.

Perception Reprogramming

Self-Examination Time. *Daily, weekly,* and *annually* reflecting on your life, your happiness, your results, and your relationships will help you to continuously improve your performance and change your belief system. When you find things are not working out, you are most likely to change direction and alter your perceptions. For the things that *are* working out, you may still alter them to make them even better—or know you should continue as you have been.

If you never change directions, you will wind up exactly where you are going. To achieve something you have never achieved before, you must do the things you have never done before. The new directions you must take and the new things you must do can be realized only through regular self-examination.

In time, your perceptions will become reprogrammed, and you will download newer, better perceptions. With a new point of view, your life can truly evolve and change.

Review Part 4: Stress Management for Your Body by God. Regularly reviewing the Stress (Peace) Management section, particularly "The 10 Instructions for Peace by God," will create more and more true understanding and improve your perceptions.

Working in Your Mission Time. Whether you get paid, do it for free, or pay someone else to allow you to do it, begin spending time in the mission for which God has chosen you. This will help improve your abilities in all the necessary areas of your mission and help move you toward accomplishing the things you love and are passionate about.

True freedom and prosperity can only come when your life's work is your mission. Then you never work another day in your life. I never say I work—I go to the joy center.

Life by God Booster #7: Just Say No! (to Stress)

It is important to do all you can to prevent yourself from ending up in a crisis mode, because if you are always in a crisis, then forget it—there is no such thing as "stress management."

At one point in my life, I had five practices, was speaking all over the country, and was taking on every new project or opportunity thrown at me. During that period, I was not effectively managing my time and did not have the right kind of delegation happening in any of my five practices. As a result, every time I left town to speak, there was a major emergency. These emergencies began to totally control my time and created a situation where everything in my life was in a crisis state. Relationship, spiritual, health, and fitness issues began popping up on a regular basis.

I lived in constant crisis for about a year and a half, with emergencies present seemingly twenty-four hours a day. As hard as I tried, the bottom line was, there was no way to manage that kind of stress. I diligently worked harder, but obviously never any smarter, because things just kept getting worse and worse.

Finally, to restore some sanity, I ended up selling the four practices in which I did not work. This made life a lot easier. Later, however, I realized the problem wasn't too many practices, it was lack of time management. Now that I am spending more Time by God, I can do considerably more than I was doing then, without a fraction of the pain and suffering.

As covered in the Stress Management portion of your manual, stress is dangerous to your body. However, the most dangerous thing about stress is that it will keep you from working in your mission and living a Life by God. That is why it is important to learn a tiny little word that will add an incredible amount of time to your schedule and eliminate a lot of emergencies . . . That word is *no*.

SETTING UP YOUR LIFE BY GOD

Paint Your Solid Yellow Lines

To start your stress-free, well-managed, unbelievably productive lives, you begin as always by painting your solid yellow lines. Paint lines around each of your lives at certain times throughout the day. Then determine what Mission-ary Work and Prosperity Times fit in each life and place those within the lines as well.

The time chart on page 340 is an example of a typical Monday in my life. Hopefully, you will see how, through proper yellow-line painting, I am able to reduce emergencies, grow spiritually, stay fit and healthy, maintain good relationships, and be successful in all areas of my mission from God. After reviewing my time chart, fill out your own on the following page for the 40-Day Plan to manage your time.

BBG Owner's Manual Guidelines for Setting Up Your Lines

1. Identify your different lives and paint solid yellow lines around them.

2. Choose the time of day you will live each life.

3. Place the Mission Work and Prosperity Times you must perform within each life in order to make it successful.

Time Chart - Dr. Ben Lerner

Morning / Afternoon

Time:	5–6am	**Time:**	6–6:45am	**Time:**	6:45–11am	**Time:**	11am–1pm	**Time:**	1pm–1:45pm

Time: 5–6am	**Time:** 6–6:45am	**Time:** 6:45–11am	**Time:** 11am–1pm	**Time:** 1pm–1:45pm
Life: Spiritual	**Life:** Author	**Life:** Doctor	**Life:** Consultant	**Life:** Health / Athlete
Missionary Work: Spiritual Growth	**Missionary Work:** Spiritual, Social, & Community	**Missionary Work:** Social & Community, Organization & Planning	**Missionary Work:** Social & Community, Organization & Planning	**Missionary Work:** Healthy Lifestyle
Prosperity Time: Prayer Time, Bible Time, Quiet Time	**Prosperity Time:** Working in mission	**Prosperity Time:** Working in Mission, Playbook Time	**Prosperity Time:** Goal-Setting Time, Playbook Time	**Special Time:** Aerobic Time

Afternoon / Evening

Time: 2–6pm	**Time:** 6–9pm	**Time:** 9–10pm	**Time:** 10pm	**Time:**
Life: Doctor	**Life:** Family	**Life:** Lecturer	**Life:** Sleep	**Life:**
Missionary Work: Relationship Building	**Missionary Work:** Relationship Building	**Missionary Work:** Opportunity, Skill Sharpening & New Skill Develop	**Missionary Work:**	**Missionary Work:**
Prosperity Time: 1 on 1 with staff, special consults w/ patients	**Prosperity Time:** Inspiration Time (books/movies)	**Prosperity Time:** Launch Time Education Time	**Prosperity Time:** Prayer Time	**Prosperity Time:**

(SYL)   (SYL)   (SYL)   (SYL)   (SYL)

SOLID YELLOW LINE (SYL)

Personal Time Chart

Morning / Afternoon

Time:	Time:	Time:	Time:	Time:
Life:	Life:	Life:	Life:	Life:
Missionary Work:	Missionary Work:	Missionary Work:	Missionary Work:	Missionary Work:
Prosperity Time:	Prosperity Time:	Prosperity Time:	Prosperity Time:	Prosperity Time:

Afternoon / Evening

Time:	Time:	Time:	Time:	Time:
Life:	Life:	Life:	Life:	Life:
Missionary Work:	Missionary Work:	Missionary Work:	Missionary Work:	Missionary Work:
Prosperity Time:	Prosperity Time:	Prosperity Time:	Prosperity Time:	Prosperity Time:

(SYL) (SYL) (SYL) (SYL)

SOLID YELLOW LINE (SYL)

23 | THE BODY BY GOD 40-DAY PLANS

Get 40 percent better for God in 40 days by improving:

Your Spirit
Your Body
Your Brain
Your Business
Your Relationships
Your Skills
And Your Outlook on Life
. . . for God.

FORGET GIVING 110 PERCENT; TRY 1 PERCENT INSTEAD

When coaches, fathers, and employers try to motivate their players, children, or staff, they often say, "Give me 110 percent!" This is the modern American way of saying 100 percent just isn't good enough anymore.

But God has something else in mind. He doesn't require 110 percent 100 percent of the time. He understands the immense challenge of caring for your BBG.

Therefore, I recommend giving 1 percent. It may not sound like much, but God—and I—understand that change is extremely difficult. That is why, by January 3, most people's New Year's resolutions have already gone the way of eight-track tapes, hula hoops, and the hustle.

If you're a smoker, you've probably tried to quit many times. If you are not happy with your weight or your waist size, you have probably begun and stopped multiple diets and exercise plans. Most likely, you have also attempted to be more positive, more outgoing, or struggled to make some other changes in your attitude and fallen short.

Why? It's not just because you're weak or unmotivated or don't know the statistics for problems associated with not taking care of your Body by God. It's because change is extremely difficult.

That is why I created the Body by God 40-Day Plans. The 40-Day Plans involve getting 1 percent better every day for 40 days. If you take small steps toward change, you can easily get 1 percent better each day. You take little baby, human steps toward God, and God will take big God steps toward you. You still may end up giving 110 percent. It just may take years.

THE BODY BY GOD "OVERNIGHT SUCCESS" ALTERNATIVE 40-DAY PLANS

Follow the *Body by God* "Overnight Success" programs found after the regular 40-Day Plans for nutrition or exercise to effect quicker, more dramatic changes in your health and appearance. Follow them together, and you will become an "overnight success."

NOTE: While stress management and time management improve with learning over time, it is possible with nutrition and exercise to see results overnight.

40 PERCENT BETTER FOR GOD IN 40 DAYS

Society has lost its health and moral compass. The people of this world are lost and, instead of walking down God's road of success, they are sprinting down the road of destruction. The reason the Body by God plan covers 40 days is that in the Bible, 40 is the number of complete and total transformation; 40 is the number of days the Bible uses for people as well as total nations to become changed, renewed, and totally revolutionized. In 40 days, you can restore "Happily Ever After."

By following the Body by God 40-Day Plans and first changing where *you* are headed, you can help God change where the *world* is headed. Like the heroes of the Bible, you can be a guide or compass that God can use to help others get back on course. That is why it is the 40-Day Plan to get better not just for yourself, but for God and everyone around you. That is your obligation, that is your direction, and that is your mission.

It is very difficult to change overnight without at some point in the future ending up right back where you started. That is why resolutions fail. You can only truly be committed to something that requires making small, steady changes. You can easily average getting 1 percent better each day for God for 40 days and continue to get 1 percent better each day (or at least each week) for the rest of your life.

The Transforming Power of 40 Days

These biblical forty-day and forty-night events altered ethical, behavioral, legal, and spiritual history forever:

- *Genesis 6–8:* Noah saw the world revolutionized by 40 days and 40 nights of rain.
- *Exodus 34:28:* Moses was with the Lord for 40 days and 40 nights when he received the Ten Commandments. To this day, the Ten Commandments are the rules at the base of all the laws and ethics we live by.
- *1 Kings 19:8:* Elijah ate one meal and did not eat again for 40 days and 40 nights, yet he had all the strength he needed to do God's work and fulfill his destiny.
- *Numbers 13:25:* The spies returned inspired and renewed after 40 days in the promised land.
- *Jonah 3:4:* Jonah foretold that Nineveh would be overturned (completely transformed) in 40 days.
- *Matthew 4:2:* Jesus fasted 40 days and 40 nights before being tempted by the devil. His holy ability to withstand the temptations of evil launched a spiritual message that would last for all eternity.
- *Acts 1:3:* Jesus presented Himself to the disciples for 40 days following His resurrection. This revealed to us that 40 days literally means full and total transformation; the death of the old and the rebirth of the new.

If it comes from God, it shouldn't be impossible to follow. It may not be totally easy, but it should come naturally and at least be semipainless. The 40-Day Plan is one that you can see yourself following for the rest of your life. It's not a cold-turkey, dive-right-in, change-everything-overnight type of program. It is making small but incredibly positive changes that in time will totally transform every facet of your life. You will look and feel better, change your overall health picture, and completely revolutionize how you look at the world you live in—all in only 40 days!

By being obedient to applying even some of the time-management techniques, nutritional rules, short Quick-Set exercise programs, and stress-management tools for changing perception, you will see how incredibly easy it is to begin making *now* the best days of your life. Living happily ever after isn't something you just read about, it is something you can experience 1 percent at a time.

Realize only God is already there. You are always *becoming* . . .

Eat for God, exercise for God, and manage your time and your stress for God. If all that sounds overwhelming, choose just one area. But begin it. There is something magical, powerful, and exciting about beginning.

> *Come near to God and he will come near to you.* (James 4:8)

THE BODY BY GOD 40-DAY PLAN FOR A LIFE BY GOD IS AS SIMPLE AS A, B, C . . . AND D

The following steps offer specific suggestions taken from your *Owner's Manual*. If you read and understand the directions, getting 40 percent better for God in 40 days really is as easy as A, B, C . . . and D.

Apply the steps below in the areas of fueling, moving, managing stress, and managing time in your BBG to completely transform your entire life in 40 days, *or simply choose one area to improve for now.* Whether you choose to improve 1 percent each day in all areas of your life or in just one or two areas, either way, you are improving for God. He loves that, He will appreciate you for it, and He will be with you every step of the way.

(A) THREE STEPS TO BECOMING 40 PERCENT BETTER AT FUELING FOR GOD IN 40 DAYS

Step #1: Implement the Addition Rule (see page 110).

Add 1 Food by God to your morning.

Examples: 1 piece of fruit, 1 bowl of oatmeal, almond butter, almond milk, vegetable omelette using 1 egg yolk and 4 egg whites, herbal tea, pure water, freshly squeezed fruit juice

Add 2 Foods by God to your midday.

Examples: vegetables, leafy salads, avocado, sweet potatoes, brown, jasmine, or basmati rice, 4 oz. (small serving) of fish, chicken breast, turkey breast, or vegetable omelette using 1 egg yolk and 4 egg whites, raw and roasted almonds, walnuts, sunflower and pumpkin seeds, herbal tea, pure water, freshly squeezed vegetable juice

Add 2 Foods by God to your evening.

Examples: vegetables, leafy salads, avocado, 6–8 oz. (large serving) of fish, chicken breast, turkey breast, olive oil-based dressing, vegetable omelette using 1 egg yolk and 4 egg whites, raw almonds, walnuts, sunflower and pumpkin seeds, herbal tea, pure water, freshly squeezed vegetable juice

Step #2: Follow the Un-Diet Food Guide.

Eat God's Way 2 Days a Week (see Food Guide on pages 82–84).

Follow the Un-Diet Food Guide 2 days each week:

- High carbohydrates, zero-low protein, low good fat in morning
- Low–moderate carbohydrates, low–moderate protein, low–moderate good fat at midday
- Very low carbohydrates (vegetables and salads only), high protein, moderate–high good fat in the evening

Step #3: Implement the Replacement and Vacation Rule (see Pages 110–14).

Use the Replacement Rule to replace 2 Foods by Man that you consume regularly or are addicted to with a healthier alternative 5 days a week. Use the Vacation Rule the other 2 days a week to eat or drink the foods you replaced.

Example #1: Use hot herb tea, hot vanilla rice milk, or chocolate almond milk 5 days a week to replace coffee. Set 2 Vacation Days aside for coffee.

Example #2: Eat fruit to replace sweets 5 days a week. Set aside 2 Vacation Days to eat a sweet that you crave.

Example #3: Use almond or rice milk to replace cow's milk 5 days a week. Set aside 2 Vacation Days for using or drinking cow's milk or doing dairy.

Get Even Better for God After 40 Days.

Follow the same plan, but continue to add more Food by God, more full days of eating God's way (using the Un-Diet Food Guide), and replace more Food by Man. *Eventually, you won't be able to imagine eating any other way!*

(B) TWO STEPS TO BECOMING 40 PERCENT BETTER AT MOVING FOR GOD IN 40 DAYS

Step #1: Add 2 Aerobic Routines.

Add 2 aerobic activities for 15+ Minutes at Fat Utilization Rate (FUR). (See: Aerobics "Moving Zones" on page 154.)

Example: 15+ minutes of jogging, biking, speed walking, inline skating, or hiking at your FUR

Step #2: Add 2 Resistance Routines.

Add 1 upper-body resistance workout and 1 lower-body resistance workout. (See: Resistance Training Programs starting on page 204.)

Example #1: One 20-minute lower-body workout and one 20-minute upper-workout using 3-Minute Body Part Quick Sets

Example #2: Two 10-minute workouts instead of one 20-minute workout using Quick Sets

Get Even Better for God After 40 Days.

Add 1 more aerobic and 1 more lower body session if you are a woman, or 1 more aerobic and 1 more upper body session if you are a man. *(Soon, missing a workout will actually bother you.)*

(C) THREE STEPS TO BECOMING 40 PERCENT BETTER AT MANAGING STRESS (CREATING PEACE) FOR GOD IN 40 DAYS

Step 1: Spiritual Growth Mission Work Every Morning.

First thing in the morning, run your 15-Minute "Spiritual Triathlon": 5 minutes of Prayer Time/5 minutes of Bible Time/5 minutes of Quiet Time. (See Prosperity Times for spiritual growth on page 326.)

Step 2: Read 2 of the "10 Instructions for Peace by God" Each Day.

(See "10 Instructions for Peace by God" on page 240.)

Step 3: 2 Mission Work Special Times Each Day.

Some examples of mission work are:

- Relationship Building—Prosperity Time: Date Time
- Social and Community—Prosperity Time: Charitable Time
- Skill Sharpening and New Skill Development—Prosperity Time: Education Time
- Organization and Planning—Prosperity Time: Playbook Time, Goal-Setting Time
- Coaching—Prosperity Time: Masterminding Time

Get Even Better for God After 40 Days.

Add 5–10 more minutes to your spiritual Triathlon-Prayer/Bible/Quiet Time, continue to read 2 of the "10 Instructions for Peace by God" every day, and continue to paint solid yellow lines around more Prosperity Times each week. *(Your stress, your outlook, and your life will transform before your eyes.)*

(D) THREE STEPS TO BECOMING 40 PERCENT BETTER AT MANAGING YOUR TIME FOR GOD IN 40 DAYS

Step 1. Define Your Different Lives.

(See "Painting Solid Yellow Lines" on page 313.)

Step 2: Paint Solid Yellow Lines Around These Lives.

Step 3: Define Work and Times.

Define the Mission Work and the Prosperity Times that must occur within it in order to make these lives successful. (See "Setting Up Your Life by God" on page 339.)

THE BODY BY GOD 40-DAY NUTRITION AND EXERCISE OVERNIGHT SUCCESS PLANS

By eating only Foods by God and following the Un-Diet program exactly as it is shown in your manual, you will very quickly see radical changes in your overall health and appearance.

Follow the Un-Diet by eliminating Food by Man and eating Food by God according to the Un-Diet Food Guide, and see a brand-new you in 40 days.

By following the "Moving Zone" and the Quick Set Program for 3-minute body parts according to the schedules for women and men described in Part 3, you can see fast, dramatic changes.

Women: Do Quick Sets for your lower body two times every 3–4 days and each muscle of your upper body every week, and turn loosely packed muscle (fat) into lean muscle.

Men: Do Quick Sets for each muscle of your upper body every 5–6 days and your lower body every week, and you can literally watch your belly shrink and your muscles grow.

Men and Women: Perform a minimum of 3 aerobic routines in the fat-burning "Moving Zones" (FUR and/or PER) each week.

By following the nutrition and exercise plans together, you can actually create unbelievable changes in your physique practically overnight. Following these two programs can make you the type of "Overnight Success" you thought could only be created through computer-enhanced "before" and "after" pictures, drugs, or plastic surgery.

Only God is perfect; you are near perfect—
but getting 1 percent better every day.

SAMPLE PLAYBOOK

(See charts on pages 353–56.)

MAKING NOW "THE GOOD OLD DAYS"

Nearly every client or patient I have ever worked with talks about "the good old days." A time long ago when they used to be in shape, used to follow an exercise program, used to read a lot, used to follow a "strict" diet, used to be a great athlete, or used to be focused on God. Apparently, at some point, "the good old days" became "the bad new now." The excuse is that their knees and backs went bad, babies were born, they got jobs, got married, or got divorced.

Most nutrition plans, exercise programs, and stress-management tools are like New Year's resolutions: They last only days. A few glorious days that many people will spend the rest of their lives remembering, saying, "I can remember when . . ." Most plans are obviously not following the 4 Rules of Olympic Success. They must be too unnatural, less than superior plans, too hard to follow, and without inspiration. If they are following the plan only for a few days, that is far from obedience to God.

If I carefully analyze my own obedience to the *Owner's Manual* plan, I see that about six times out of ten, I do not necessarily feel like following it. More than half the time, I am not overly motivated to put in my Bible Time, Nutrition Time, Education Time, Exercise Time, and all the other times necessary to attain and keep my Life by God. The reason I usually *do* follow the plan and have been doing good things for my BBG consistently for years is that, although I do not always feel like doing it, I am inspired to do it anyway—no excuses!

As a result, now is "the good old days."

WHAT IS THE MEANING OF LIFE?

I have heard it said, "Life is one darn thing after another." I, however, have found it to be more than that—a *great* deal more.

When you have a birthday and someone asks you if you feel any older, well, you pretty much feel like you did the day before. Birth*days*, holi*days*, Mon*days*, Sun*days*, or any *days* always feel the same or similar to the day before. But they are not. What each day represents is another chance at "it." Another chance at doing things better than you did the year, month, week, or day before. A better chance at having a higher-quality day, a more moral day, a healthier day, a more joyful day, a day in which you are more loving to others, and a day in which you are better for God then the day before.

Your path is not about reaching the summit of a mountain, a final destination, or getting to the last target. Your path is about continuous development and always moving up the mountain. Life is a never-ending story in which you are constantly opening windows, breaking through the clouds, and watching the sunrise.

Only God is perfect. You are not looking for perfect. You will have faults, and you will make mistakes. However, as long as you are always in a state of perpetual growth, you are a "work in progress."

You are not perfect; you are "near perfect." You would not want to reach perfect, even if it were possible, because once you are perfect you can only get worse. Once a tomato is ripe, it begins to rot. You are not perfect, but that is okay—as long as you are working on it. All you can do is the very best you can do. The outcome of your life is ultimately not up to you. It is up to God.

As you continue to work on getting 1 percent better for God each day, often you will not get the results you had hoped or planned to receive. Just keep remembering that perpetual growth and faithful action are your job; the results are His. As you continue to keep trying to do the things you know to be right, an unfortunate but very common occurrence is that you will get discouraged or make errors. At these times, do not quit. Just get back to simply getting 1 percent better for God. When you make mistakes, remember, only God is perfect. You are only "near perfect," but you are working on it.

**Only the divinely wise and the totally ignorant
shall not get 1 percent better for God . . .**

PLEASE SHARE YOUR RESULTS!

Keep a journal of how your life changes along the course of the 40-Day Plan. Record the emotional changes, stress reduction, relationship improvements, and family and financial successes that all occur in your new Life by God.

Take before and after photos and measurements of your weight and your waist, arm, chest, and thigh sizes to see the effects of the Food by God and Exercise by God programs.

Send us a copy of your pictures, measurements, and a short story of how you got 40 percent better for God (or some percentage for God) in only 40 days.

Many blessings,

Dr. Ben

To send in your results and/or for more information on Body by God products, services, providing doctors, and/or to contact Dr. Ben, visit:

www.thebodybygod.com.

Personal BBG 40-Day Plan Playbook

MONDAY

Time:	Time:	Time:	Time:	Time:	Time:	Time:	Time:	Time:	Time:
Life:	Life:	Life:	Life:	Life:	Life:	Life:	Life:	Life:	Life:
Missionary Work:	Missionary Work:	Missionary Work:	Missionary Work:	Missionary Work:	Missionary Work:	Missionary Work:	Missionary Work:	Missionary Work:	Missionary Work:
Special Time:	Special Time:	Special Time:	Special Time:	Special Time:	Special Time:	Special Time:	Special Time:	Special Time:	Special Time:

(SYL) (SYL) (SYL) (SYL) (SYL) (SYL) (SYL) (SYL) (SYL)

SOLID YELLOW LINE (SYL)

TUESDAY

Time:	Time:	Time:	Time:	Time:	Time:	Time:	Time:	Time:	Time:
Life:	Life:	Life:	Life:	Life:	Life:	Life:	Life:	Life:	Life:
Missionary Work:	Missionary Work:	Missionary Work:	Missionary Work:	Missionary Work:	Missionary Work:	Missionary Work:	Missionary Work:	Missionary Work:	Missionary Work:
Special Time:	Special Time:	Special Time:	Special Time:	Special Time:	Special Time:	Special Time:	Special Time:	Special Time:	Special Time:

(SYL) (SYL) (SYL) (SYL) (SYL) (SYL) (SYL) (SYL) (SYL)

SOLID YELLOW LINE (SYL)

Personal BBG 40-Day Plan Playbook

WEDNESDAY

Time:	Time:	Time:	Time:	Time:	Time:	Time:	Time:	Time:	Time:
Life:	Life:	Life:	Life:	Life:	Life:	Life:	Life:	Life:	Life:
Missionary Work:	Missionary Work:	Missionary Work:	Missionary Work:	Missionary Work:	Missionary Work:	Missionary Work:	Missionary Work:	Missionary Work:	Missionary Work:
Special Time:	Special Time:	Special Time:	Special Time:	Special Time:	Special Time:	Special Time:	Special Time:	Special Time:	Special Time:

(SYL) (SYL) (SYL) (SYL) (SYL) (SYL) (SYL) (SYL) (SYL)

SOLID YELLOW LINE (SYL)

THURSDAY

Time:	Time:	Time:	Time:	Time:	Time:	Time:	Time:	Time:	Time:
Life:	Life:	Life:	Life:	Life:	Life:	Life:	Life:	Life:	Life:
Missionary Work:	Missionary Work:	Missionary Work:	Missionary Work:	Missionary Work:	Missionary Work:	Missionary Work:	Missionary Work:	Missionary Work:	Missionary Work:
Special Time:	Special Time:	Special Time:	Special Time:	Special Time:	Special Time:	Special Time:	Special Time:	Special Time:	Special Time:

(SYL) (SYL) (SYL) (SYL) (SYL) (SYL) (SYL) (SYL) (SYL)

SOLID YELLOW LINE (SYL)

Personal BBG 40-Day Plan Playbook

FRIDAY

Time:	Time:	Time:	Time:	Time:	Time:	Time:	Time:	Time:	Time:
Life:	Life:	Life:	Life:	Life:	Life:	Life:	Life:	Life:	Life:
Missionary Work:	Missionary Work:	Missionary Work:	Missionary Work:	Missionary Work:	Missionary Work:	Missionary Work:	Missionary Work:	Missionary Work:	Missionary Work:
Special Time:	Special Time:	Special Time:	Special Time:	Special Time:	Special Time:	Special Time:	Special Time:	Special Time:	Special Time:

(SYL) (SYL) (SYL) (SYL) (SYL) (SYL) (SYL) (SYL) (SYL)

SOLID YELLOW LINE (SYL)

SATURDAY

Time:	Time:	Time:	Time:	Time:	Time:	Time:	Time:	Time:	Time:
Life:	Life:	Life:	Life:	Life:	Life:	Life:	Life:	Life:	Life:
Missionary Work:	Missionary Work:	Missionary Work:	Missionary Work:	Missionary Work:	Missionary Work:	Missionary Work:	Missionary Work:	Missionary Work:	Missionary Work:
Special Time:	Special Time:	Special Time:	Special Time:	Special Time:	Special Time:	Special Time:	Special Time:	Special Time:	Special Time:

(SYL) (SYL) (SYL) (SYL) (SYL) (SYL) (SYL) (SYL) (SYL)

SOLID YELLOW LINE (SYL)

Personal BBG 40-Day Plan Playbook

SUNDAY

Time:	Time:	Time:	Time:	Time:	Time:	Time:	Time:
Life:	Life:	Life:	Life:	Life:	Life:	Life:	Life:
Missionary Work:	Missionary Work:	Missionary Work:	Missionary Work:	Missionary Work:	Missionary Work:	Missionary Work:	Missionary Work:
Special Time:	Special Time:	Special Time:	Special Time:	Special Time:	Special Time:	Special Time:	Special Time:
(SYL)	(SYL)	(SYL)	(SYL)	(SYL)	(SYL)	(SYL)	(SYL)

SOLID YELLOW LINE (SYL)

EXTRA *BODY BY GOD* CHARTS AND FORMS

MORNING BODY BY GOD UN-DIET Nutrient Evaluation Form

Date	Real Time	Intended Time by God
....	.... A.M./P.M.	.... A.M./P.M.

Actual Food | Why You Ate/Drank? | Planned Food by God

Actual Food		Planned Food by God
Carbohydrate:		Carbohydrate:
Protein:		Protein:
Fat:		Fat:
Liquid:		Liquid:
Food by Man:		Food by Man:
How you felt after eating	How you felt 1-2 hours later	

MIDDAY | BODY BY GOD UN-DIET | Nutrient Evaluation Form

Date	Real Time	Intended Time by God
	A.M./P.M.	A.M./P.M.

Actual Food | Why You Ate/Drank? | Planned Food by God

Carbohydrate:

Protein:

Fat:

Liquid:

Food by Man:

How you felt after eating

How you felt 1-2 hours later

Carbohydrate:

Protein:

Fat:

Liquid:

Food by Man:

EVENING

BODY BY GOD UN-DIET — Nutrient Evaluation Form

Date	Real Time	Intended Time by God
....	.... A.M./P.M.	.... A.M./P.M.

Actual Food

Carbohydrate:

Protein:

Fat:

Liquid:

Food by Man:

How you felt after eating

Why You Ate/Drank?

Planned Food by God

Carbohydrate:

Protein:

Fat:

Liquid:

Food by Man:

How you felt 1-2 hours later

PERSONAL AEROBIC ROUTINES

30-Minute Cardiovascular Movement
(+10 MINUTE WARM-UP/COOLDOWN = 40 MINUTE TOTAL)

FOR FAT BURNING

WARNING - Before you begin: Never start an exercise program without first consulting your physician. Those with a personal history of heart disease, high blood pressure, high cholesterol, cancer, diabetes, or who smoke or are overweight should begin exercising with professional supervision.

Name: _____

Age: _____ Gender: _____

ACTIVITY: _____

FUR - Fat-Utilization Rate

PER - Performance Enhancement Rate

SUR - Sugar-Utilization Rate

FUR: _____ PER: _____ SUR: _____

MOVING ZONE LEVELS				
TIME (Elapsed)	TIME (Per Stage)	HEART RATE	SPEED/INCLINE OR LEVEL/RPM	HEART RATE (Real)
0:00	0:00	Resting Heart Rate (RHR)+	Mph/	RHR
5:00	5:00	Below - FUR	Mph/	
7:00	2:00	Near - FUR	Mph/	
9:00	2:00	Nearer - FUR	Mph/	
14:00	5:00	First 1% - FUR	Mph/	
19:00	5:00	First 10% - FUR	Mph/	
24:00	5:00	First 50% - FUR	Mph/	
29:00	5:00	First 10% - FUR	Mph/	
32:00	3:00	First 1% - FUR	Mph/	
35:00	3:00	Near - FUR	Mph/	
40:00	5:00	Below - FUR - RHR+	Mph/	

PERSONAL AEROBIC ROUTINES

40-Minute Cardiovascular Movement
(+10 minute warm-up/cooldown= 50 minute total)

FOR FAT BURNING AND IMPROVED PERFORMANCE

Name: _____

Age: _____ Gender: _____

ACTIVITY: _____

WARNING - Before you begin: Never start an exercise program without first consulting your physician. Those with a personal history of heart disease, high blood pressure, high cholesterol, cancer, diabetes, or who smoke or are overweight should begin exercising with professional supervision.

FUR - Fat-Utilization Rate PER - Performance Enhancement Rate SUR - Sugar-Utilization Rate

FUR: _____ PER: _____ SUR: _____

| MOVING ZONE LEVELS | | | | |
TIME (Elapsed)	TIME (Per Stage)	HEART RATE	SPEED/INCLINE OR LEVEL/RPM	HEART RATE (Real)
0:00	0:00	Resting Heart Rate (RHR)+	0 Mph/ 0	
5:00	5:00	Below - FUR	Mph/	
7:00	2:00	Near - FUR	Mph/	
9:00	2:00	Nearer - FUR	Mph/	
11:00	2:00	First 1% - FUR	Mph/	
13:00	2:00	First 10% - FUR	Mph/	
15:00	2:00	First 10% - FUR	Mph/	
18:00	3:00	First 50% - FUR	Mph/	
21:00	3:00	Last 50% - FUR	Mph/	
25:00	4:00	First 50% - PER	Mph/	
29:00	4:00	First 50% - PER	Mph/	
33:00	4:00	Last 50% - PER	Mph/	
36:00	3:00	Last 50% - PER	Mph/	
39:00	3:00	PER - FUR	Mph/	
42:00	3:00	Last 50% - FUR	Mph/	
45:00	3:00	First 50% - FUR	Mph/	
50:00	5:00	First 10% - FUR - RHR +	Mph/	

PERSONAL AEROBIC ROUTINES

40-MINUTE CARDIOVASCULAR MOVEMENT
(+10 MINUTE WARM-UP/COOLDOWN= 50 MINUTE TOTAL)

FOR FAT BURNING AND SPORTS/PEAK PERFORMANCE

Name: _____

Age: _____ Gender: _____

ACTIVITY: _____

FUR - Fat-Utilization Rate   **PER** - Performance Enhancement Rate   **SUR** - Sugar-Utilization Rate

FUR: _____   PER: _____   SUR: _____

MOVING ZONE LEVELS				
TIME (Elapsed)	**TIME** (Per Stage)	**HEART RATE**	**SPEED/INCLINE OR LEVEL/RPM**	**HEART RATE** (Real)
0:00	0:00	Resting Heart Rate+	0Mph 0	
5:00	5:00	Below - FUR	Mph	
7:00	2:00	Near - FUR	Mph	
9:00	2:00	Nearer - FUR	Mph	
11:00	2:00	First 1% - FUR	Mph	
13:00	2:00	First 50% - FUR	Mph	
15:00	2:00	First 50% - PER	Mph	
17:00	2:00	SUR	Mph	
19:00	2:00	PER - FUR	Mph	
21:00	2:00	PER	Mph	
24:00	3:00	SUR	Mph	
26:00	2:00	PER - FUR	Mph	
28:00	2:00	PER	Mph	
32:00	4:00	SUR	Mph	
34:00	2:00	PER - FUR	Mph	
36:00	2:00	PER	Mph	
41:00	5:00	SUR	Mph	
45:00	4:00	PER - FUR	Mph	
50:00	5:00	FUR - RHR+	Mph	

The Daily BBG Fitness Program

Body Parts: ....

Real Date	Real Time	Intended Date	Intended Time by God
——	.... A.M./P.M.		.... A.M./P.M.

Types of Sets

Legs:
Upper Body:

•Decline - **D**	•Pause - **P**	•Mountain - **M**	•Cycle - **C**	•Monster Set - **MO**
15 - 5 reps	12 - 0 reps	15 - 5 reps	15 - 6 reps	
12 - 5 reps	12 - 0 reps	12 - 5 reps	12 - 6 reps	

Movements

	Type of Set					Real		Intended	
Lower Body Movements	D	P	M	C	MO	Reps	Weight	Reps	Weight

10 Minutes   20 Minutes   30 Minutes

The Daily BBG Fitness Program

Body Parts: _____

Real Date	Real Time	Intended Date	Intended Time by God
	.... A.M./P.M.		.... A.M./P.M.

Types of Sets

Legs:	•Decline - **D**	•Pause - **P**	•Mountain - **M**	•Cycle - **C**	•Monster Set - **MO**
	15 - 5 reps	12 - 0 reps	15 - 5 reps	15 - 6 reps	
Upper Body:	12 - 5 reps	12 - 0 reps	12 - 5 reps	12 - 6 reps	

Movements	Type of Set				Real			Intended	
Upper-Body Movements	D	P	M	C	MO	Reps	Weight	Reps	Weight

10 Minutes   20 Minutes   30 Minutes

Generalized Personal Time Chart

MORNING/AFTERNOON

Time:	Time:	Time:	Time:
Life:	Life:	Life:	Life:

AFTERNOON/EVENING

Time:	Time:	Time:	Time:
Life:	Life:	Life:	Life:

(SYL)   (SYL)   (SYL)   (SYL)

SOLID YELLOW LINE (SYL)

Personal Time Chart

Morning / Afternoon

Time:	Time:	Time:	Time:
Life:	Life:	Life:	Life:
Missionary Work:	Missionary Work:	Missionary Work:	Missionary Work:
Prosperity Time:	Prosperity Time:	Prosperity Time:	Prosperity Time:

Afternoon / Evening

Time:	Time:	Time:	Time:
Life:	Life:	Life:	Life:
Missionary Work:	Missionary Work:	Missionary Work:	Missionary Work:
Prosperity Time:	Prosperity Time:	Prosperity Time:	Prosperity Time:

(SYL)   (SYL)   (SYL)   (SYL)

SOLID YELLOW LINE (SYL)

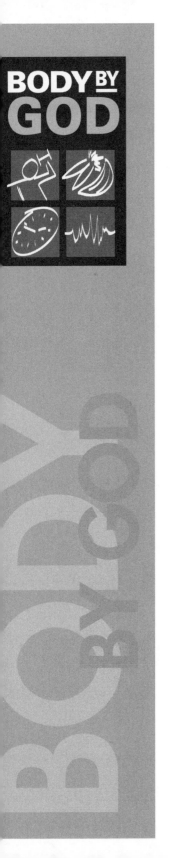

Check out the Body By God website today to:

- Find the latest information on nutrition, movement, peace management, time management, relationships, and prosperity.

- Sign up for the eNewsletter that will bring the latest in maximized living straight to your mailbox twice a week.

- Find answers to commonly asked questions.

- Learn how you can get Dr. Ben or a Body by God provider in your area to hold a seminar or workshop.

- Find a Body by God practitioner in your area.

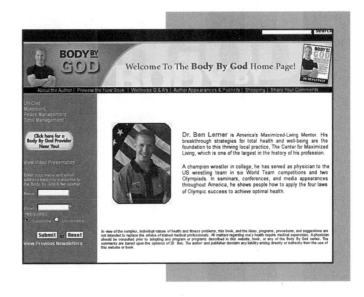

www.thebodybygod.com